SPORT FOR LIFE

AEROBIC DANCE

Phyllis C. Jacobson
Brigham Young University

BOWLING

Joyce M. Harrison
Brigham Young University
Ron Maxey

CYCLING

Lee N. Burkett
Paul W. Darst
Arizona State University

GOLF

James Ewers
University of Utah

JOGGING

David E. Corbin
*University of Nebraska
at Omaha*

KARATE

Richard J. Schmidt
*University of Nebraska
at Lincoln*
James L. Hesson
Delta State University

RACQUETBALL

Robert P. Pangrazi
Arizona State University

STRENGTH TRAINING
Beginners, Bodybuilders, and Athletes

Philip E. Allsen
Brigham Young University

TENNIS

Anne M. Pittman
Arizona State University

Charles B. Corbin/Philip E. Allsen, Series Editors

AEROBIC DANCE

Phyllis C. Jacobson
Brigham Young University

Charles B. Corbin/Philip E. Allsen, Series Editors

Scott, Foresman and Company
Glenview, Illinois   Boston   London

Cover photograph by Robert Drea

Figures 2.1–2.2 and Tables 2.1–2.2 reprinted by permission of Hooked on Aerobics, Inc.

Tables A.1–A.2 courtesy of Metropolitan Life Insurance Company.

Tables A.3–A.7 from *Physiology of Fitness* by Brian J. Sharkey. © 1979. Reprinted by permission of Human Kinetics Publishers, Inc., Champaign, Il.

Tables A.8–A.9 from *The Aerobics Program for Total Well-Being* by Kenneth Cooper. © 1983. Reprinted by permission of Bantam Books, Inc.

Library of Congress Cataloging-in-Publication Data

Jacobson, Phyllis C.
    Aerobic dance / Phyllis C. Jacobson.
        p.   cm. — (Sport for life)
    Bibliography: p.
    Includes index.
    ISBN 0-673-18522-2 (soft)
    1. Aerobic dancing. I. Title. II. Series: Sport for life
series.
RA781.15.J33 1988
613.7'1—dc 19   88-14142
                                                        CIP

ISBN 0-673-18522-2

1 2 3 4 5 6 7—MAL—93 92 91 90 89 88

Foreword

We are calling this series SPORT FOR LIFE because we believe a sports skills series should be more than just a presentation of the "rules of the game." A popular sport or activity should be presented in a way that encourages understanding through direct experience, improvement through prompt correction, and enjoyment through proper mental attitude.

Over the years, each SPORT FOR LIFE author has instructed thousands of people in their selected activity. We are delighted these "master teachers" have agreed to put down in writing the concepts and procedures they have developed successfully in teaching a skill.

The books in the SPORT FOR LIFE Series present other unique features as appropriate to the featured sport or activity.

The Sport Experience: This is a learning activity that explains and teaches a technique or specific rule. Whether it requires the reader to experience selecting a specific bicycle, stroking a backhand in tennis, or choosing an approach to use in bowling it carries the learner right to the heart of the game or activity at a pace matching his or her own progress. The Sport Experience is identified throughout the book with its own special typographical design.

The Error Corrector: The SPORT FOR LIFE authors have taken specific skills and listed some of the common errors encountered by participants; at the same time they have listed the methods to be utilized to correct these errors. The Error Corrector can be compared to a road map as it provides checkpoints toward skillful performance of a sport or activity.

The Mental Game: Understanding the mental game can remove many of the obstacles to success. The authors have devised techniques to aid the reader in planning playing strategy and in learning how to cope with the stress of competition. It is just as important to know how to remove mental errors as it is to deal with the physical ones.

The editors and authors of SPORT FOR LIFE trust that their approach and enthusiasm will have a lasting effect on each reader and will help promote a lifetime of health and happiness, physically and psychologically, for a sport well played or an activity well performed.

Charles B. Corbin/Philip E. Allsen

About the Author and Editors

Phyllis C. Jacobson. Dr. Jacobson is Chairman of the Brigham Young University Department of Physical Education–Dance. Broadly experienced as a teacher, coach, and fitness consultant, she has received numerous awards, including the Honor Award of the American Alliance of Health, Physical Education, Recreation and Dance, in recognition of her contributions. Author of many books and articles on fitness, Dr. Jacobson has also created and designed the popular T.V. series "Hooked on Aerobics." She holds a number of professional offices in the field of physical education and has served on the National Olympic Planning Committee and as speaker and consultant in aerobic dance.

Charles B. Corbin. Dr. Corbin is Professor of Physical Education at Arizona State University. A widely known expert on fitness and health, he is author or coauthor of 27 books addressed to students on those topics ranging from the elementary school through college. In August 1986, he was given the "Better Health and Living Award" by that magazine as one of ten Americans who have made the difference in influencing others in the areas of health and fitness. He is a 1982 recipient of the National Honor Award from the American Alliance for Health, Physical Education, Recreation and Dance and is a fellow in the American Academy of Physical Education.

Philip E. Allsen. Dr. Allsen is Professor of Physical Education and Director of the Fitness for Life Program at Brigham Young University in Provo, Utah. Widely known for his expertise in physical fitness, sports medicine, and athletic training, Dr. Allsen, a prolific writer, has authored more than 75 articles and written six books covering the topics of strength and physical fitness. The "Fitness for Life" program, which Dr. Allsen developed at Brigham Young University, now serves approximately 7,000 students at the institution each year, and has been adopted by more than 400 schools in the United States. He is a member of the American College of Sports Medicine; the American Alliance of Health, Physical Education, Recreation and Dance; and the National Collegiate Physical Education Association.

Preface

Aerobic Dance has been written for the novice, the occasional participant, and the highly conditioned aerobic performer. It provides dy-
namic, versatile exercise programs that can be tailored to your
individual skill and fitness level.

The first three chapters describe the benefits of aerobic dance,
how to prepare for it, and how to use the Goal Setting Chart to set
goals that are realistic for you. Then, using the numerous photographs
and sample routines, you'll learn warm-up exercises, arm movements,
and both smooth-impact and soft-rebound skills. You'll soon be cho-
reographing your own routines.

Throughout the book, "The Aerobic Experience" describes prac-
tical activities that get you into aerobic dance at your own pace, and
the skill tables help you to do so safely and efficiently. In the appen-
dixes, you'll find tests for assessing your strength, endurance, and
flexibility.

Creator of the popular PBS series "Hooked on Aerobics," the author has had the opportunity to supervise aerobic exercise programs for
thousands of people. *Aerobic Dance* brings together her knowledge and
experience to help you develop your personal routines for a lifetime of
fitness.

Acknowledgments

I would like to offer my sincere appreciation to Virginia Lee Miner and
Karen Pierotti, typists; Claudia Hill, Courtney Ekins, Jennifer Hicks,
Cheryl Hansen, Nancy Barger, Steve Gray, and Steve Turnbull, mod-
els; and Mark Philbrick, photographer.

Contents

Why Do Aerobic Dance?

Fifteen years ago, the term *aerobic dance* was known to very few people. Dr. Kenneth H. Cooper was conducting tests to measure aerobic capacity (the efficiency of the heart and lungs in processing oxygen) when the vivacious former cheerleader Jacki Sorensen volunteered to be a subject. Jacki was a dancer, not a runner, as were most of those who achieved the "excellent" rating in the test for aerobic capacity. Jacki coupled the term *dance* with *aerobic* and started a program for fitness based on traditional songleader-style dance movements.

WHAT IS AEROBIC DANCE?

Aerobic dance can best be defined as continuous movement—exercise, locomotor movement, and dance steps—performed to music. The variety and style of the movement and the musical accompaniment provide as many forms of aerobic dance programs as there are interests and tastes of people performing them. In contrast to a competitive or solitary fitness program, aerobic dance provides an opportunity for people of widely different levels of physical ability to participate together in the same facility, with the same musical accompaniment, engaging in exercises and skills which have been choreographed according to the needs of each individual.

THE FOUR PHASES OF AN
AEROBIC DANCE WORKOUT

An aerobic dance workout is divided into four phases: warm-up, skill review, aerobic, and cool-down. Each phase has its own purposes, without which the workout is incomplete. Each phase of the program is necessary if aerobic dance is to provide the desired benefits.

Warm-up Phase

The purpose of the warm-up is to do the following:

1. Prepare your body for vigorous exercise. This is done by engaging in light movement to increase blood circulation (and thus the supply of nutrients) to every muscle group. A variety of arm movements are done while basic footwork is performed.
2. Prevent stress, stiffness, pain, and injury during the vigorous aerobic phase. A proper warm-up includes sustained stretching of the major muscle groups to increase flexibility (do not bob, bounce, or jerk on a stretched muscle) and increased resistance to strengthen muscles.
3. Increase performance ability. A proper warm-up will prepare you physically and psychologically to perform at a more efficient and skillful level.

Skill-Review Phase

The first routine should be a review of skills (progressing from low to high) to gradually raise the heart rate to within your personal training zone (see PTZ charts, Chapter 2) and a review of the skills to be performed in the aerobic workout.

Aerobic Workout Phase

The aerobic phase is designed to strengthen the heart and lungs and all other body systems. To maximize the benefits, stay within the PTZ. In addition to increasing health and well-being, you will increase body-movement skills and enjoy the experience of this phase.

The skills included for the aerobic sections of the program are of two styles: *smooth impact* and *soft rebound.* When performing smooth-impact movements, the performer always has one foot on the floor; and the intensity is varied by bending the knees deeper and extending further into the movement.

On the other hand, the soft-rebound style is characterized by skills that are combinations or variations of the locomotor skills of walking, running, hopping, jumping, leaping, galloping, skipping, and sliding. Each of these basic skills can be performed at varying speed and intensity. The term *soft rebound* is descriptive of the skill. "Rebound" indicates that you will take-off and land, and "soft" indicates the quality of the landing.

Cool-Down Phase

The last, or cool-down, phase of the workout simply involves moving at a slower pace until your heart rate has returned to near normal. The action of the muscles helps the heart circulate the blood. If you stop immediately after a vigorous workout, you may become nauseated, dizzy, or faint or suffer other forms of illness. So in the cool-down phase, you continue to move at a progressively slower and lower effort level for a three- to five-minute cool-down routine. You then perform sustained stretching and resistance exercises to increase flexibility and strength of the muscles. Finally, you end with a few moments of relaxation to prepare you to engage in your daily scheduled activities with complete control and sufficient energy for success.

Further benefits of the cool-down are an increase in skeletal muscle strength and endurance, which can reduce common strain and pain, such as aching back and legs; an increase in flexibility, which can reduce strain and pain associated with stiffness of the muscles and joints; and an increase in the efficiency of body systems, with signs of degeneration and aging decreasing.

THE BENEFITS OF AEROBIC DANCE

The best reason to start aerobic dancing is that it's fun: you can tailor-make your workout to music you like, with friends you enjoy. But aerobic dance also affords each participant the benefits of all components of fitness, including flexibility, strength, cardiovascular endurance, agility, balance, and coordination. Through strengthening exercises, the muscles become better defined, and your body becomes firmer and more attractively contoured. By strengthening the muscles, you are able to achieve correct body alignment and body carriage. With increased flexibility and strength, you are able to move with freedom, rhythm, and grace. The soft rebound skills increase your balance and coordination, which carry over to many other sports and everyday activities. And with increased energy and signs of vitality, you take on a healthy, vibrant appearance.

But not only do you *look* healthier, you *feel* healthier and you *are* healthier!

The heart becomes stronger and more effective as a pump, resulting in a slower resting heart rate and a smaller increase in exercise heart rate for a given amount of work. The strength and endurance of the respiratory muscles increase, resulting in an increase of the interior volume of the lungs. Consequently, more interior surface is available for the exchange of gases with the circulatory systems, a gain which allows you to exercise longer and at a higher intensity before becoming fatigued. The capillaries—the tiny blood vessels that deliver nutrients to tissues—increase in number and provide more surface area for the exchange of oxygen and carbon dioxide between the blood and cells. This increase in capillaries also speeds up the rate of exchange of nutrients for the waste products of cell metabolism, so the efficiency of food digestion and waste elimination is increased.

A regular program of aerobic dance can lay the foundation for an invigorated, enriched, healthy life. No matter what your present fitness level—a novice, a "sometime" exerciser, or a highly conditioned longtime performer—if you enjoy music and movement and seek a higher degree of physical conditioning, aerobic dance may soon become your favorite form of exercise.

In this book you will learn what to wear when you do aerobic dance. More important, you will learn how to assess your present physical fitness level so that you can do the movements, develop the skills, and create the dance routines that will best meet your fitness needs. And you will learn specific warm-up, cool-down, soft-rebound, and smooth-impact skills that constitute aerobic dance routines. Get ready to join the thousands of men and women of all ages and fitness levels who have already enjoyed the fun—and the benefits—of this fastest-growing form of physical exercise!

Getting Started

Before beginning an aerobic dance program, review the following measures designed to prevent injury and ensure the success of a regular and long-range fitness program.

Where and When?

1. Schedule your time to participate three or four days each week. A regular schedule of exercise is important; make it a lifetime practice.
2. Perform on a wood or carpet-over-wood floor. Do not exercise on cement, carpet over cement, or tile. These surfaces cause pain and joint trauma.

Dealing with Physical Limitations

3. If you are over thirty-five years of age or have been ill or inactive, have your doctor advise you on starting a fitness program.
4. If you are obese or need support to help keep your balance, sit on a chair and move your arms, legs, torso—all muscles over which you have control—or hold on to a chair, windowsill, table top, or other stable frame.
5. If you use a walker for support, follow the instructions at the low level, doing as many skills as possible.
6. If you are in a wheelchair, in bed, or otherwise confined, move any

part of your body you are able to move. Start at a low level and progress slowly, but do get started. Devise exercises that you can do.

What to Wear

7. Wear properly fitted shoes that have cushioned soles which slide easily on the floor, a good arch support, a support for lateral movement, and a firm heel. Many shoes on the market meet these standards. Wear shoes that fit your foot to give you the best support. Shoes traditionally designed for running are not recommended for aerobic dance because of the rough textured surface of the sole and the lack of support for lateral movement.
8. Wear socks to absorb perspiration and to protect your skin from the inner surface of the shoe.
9. Wear loose-fitting activity clothes for freedom of movement (shirt and shorts, exercise suit, leotards and tights, etc.).

Being Aware of Your Needs

10. Begin any new activity at a low level and gradually progress to a higher level.
11. Be aware of pain. It is your body's indication that stress and strain exist and that continued activity may result in acute or chronic injury.
12. Follow the level that is just right for you. Follow the instructions and make the appropriate skill and intensity adjustments.

Individual differences are important. It is very unlikely that any two people are at the exact same fitness level. Therefore, to gain the benefits without undue stress and strain, you must engage in a fitness program that is designed for *you*, based on *your* present fitness level, and at a progression that enables *you* to reach *your* highest potential.

The material in this book is presented in the format of the popular *Hooked on Aerobics* television series created by this author. This is to better meet the needs of participants ranging in age from children to octogenarians and varying in movement skills from the novice to the professional and in fitness from the very poor to excellent. The designated low-, medium-, and high-intensity levels with variations in skill from one level to the other allow each participant to engage in a progressive resistance program to reach and maintain fitness for enriched, healthy living.

GOAL SETTING

Each body has specific weaknesses and strengths. Before you can improve fitness—lessen the weaknesses while maintaining and enhancing strengths—you must make a careful assessment to determine the best program for you to obtain optimum fitness and well-being. Appendix A includes tests for five standards of fitness: resting heart rate, muscular strength and endurance, flexibility, cardiovascular fitness, and lean body mass (ratio of muscle mass to fat). With information based on your assessments of these standards, you can decide what your individual strengths and weaknesses are and where you would like to improve. You may be flexible in the shoulders but have short hamstrings. You may have strong legs but weak shoulders and arms. You may be at a high level in cardiovascular fitness but lack flexibility in major muscle groups. Whatever your needs, you can study the skill section of this book and determine goals that are realistic for you—short-range as well as long-range goals to help you individualize your aerobic conditioning program.

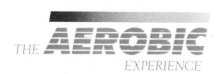

THE AEROBIC
EXPERIENCE

PROGRESS TO FITNESS

1. See the Progress to Fitness goal sheet, Figure 2.1. Write your goals down; be specific about the target you want to reach and the activities you will do to help you reach it. For example:
    I will be able to

    a. do five more pushups
    b. do ten more abdominal curls

Figure 2.1 Progress to Fitness: Goal Setting

Goal
Target Date—I will reach my goal on or before _____
Obstacles and Roadblocks—These stand between me and my goals:
Solutions and Plans—I will overcome obstacles by taking these actions:
Expected Benefits—Reaching this goal will benefit me in these ways:
Is It Worth It to Me?—Am I willing to invest this time and effort to obtain the expected benefits _____ yes _____ no

Progress Report—My progress rating on the date indicated:

Date _____	Poor ____	Fair ____	Good ____	Excellent ____
Date _____	Poor ____	Fair ____	Good ____	Excellent ____
Date _____	Poor ____	Fair ____	Good ____	Excellent ____
Date _____	Poor ____	Fair ____	Good ____	Excellent ____

Motivational ideas to help me reach my goals:

Goal Achieved

Date of achievement _____

Comments about my experience that will help me achieve
additional goals:

c. increase flexibility in each area by at least one inch
  d. trim a quarter inch of fatty tissue from abdomen
  e. lower resting heart rate by three beats

2. Set a realistic date of ten to twelve weeks. Write this date on your goal sheet under "target date."

3. Analyze the obstacles and roadblocks you will need to overcome to achieve your goals. Do you need to schedule a specific, regular time for your aerobic dance workout? Do you need to find friends with whom to work out, to motivate you? Write these problems—and their solutions—down.

4. List the benefits you will receive when you reach your goals.

5. Your commitment to invest the time and effort necessary to reach your goals depends on how much you value good health, improved appearance, increased energy, and a better lifestyle.

6. Monitor your progress by testing yourself at intervals of from eight to ten weeks.

7. Write down reminders you can use to encourage yourself along the road to reaching your goals. Success encourages you to continue.

8. Evaluate your progress or lack of progress when you have reached your target date. This is also a good time to set additional goals.

HOW HARD DO YOU NEED TO EXERCISE TO REACH A TRAINING EFFECT?

Physiologists have found that each person needs to work at least 60 percent of his or her personal maximum for a training effect to take place. They have also recommended that, for best results, no one exceed 80 percent of his or her personal maximum.

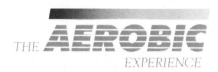

FIND YOUR PERSONAL TRAINING ZONE *(PTZ)*

Look at the Personal Training Zone Charts, Figure 2.2, and follow these directions to determine the upper and lower limits of your PTZ:

1. Find the number along the bottom of the chart that corresponds to your age.
2. Follow that line upward till it intersects (a) the line representing 60 percent of maximum heart rate—the rate at which you should work to have a training effect; or (b) the diagonal representing 70 percent of maximum heart rate—a medium level; or (c) the diagonal representing 80 percent of maximum heart rate—the upper limit that you cannot safely exceed in your program. Exceptions are limited to highly conditioned persons.
3. Stay within your PTZ. You should become sensitive to your own body and exercise at the intensity that is neither too light nor too demanding. If your program is too light, you will not see progress and, consequently, will lose interest. However, if your program is too demanding, you may suffer from the following symptoms: (a) your heart and respiration rates failing to return to normal within 15 minutes after a vigorous, strenuous workout; (b) disturbed rest and sleep; (c) a feeling of tiredness or depression the day after exercising; (d) muscle soreness and stiffness.

    Note: A medium-intensity level is more effective than a high-intensity level if you wish to trim fat from your body.

Table 2.1 will help you convert your 10-second exercise heart rate to 1-minute rate. Table 2.2 will help you establish your lower and upper limits, based on your age and your 10-second exercise heart rate.

Figure 2.2 PTZ Charts (RHR–75)

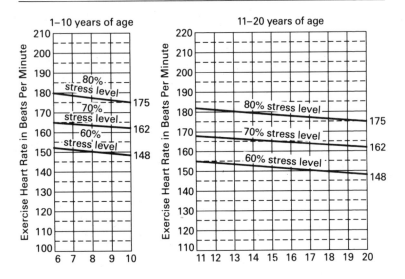

1–10 years of age

11–20 years of age

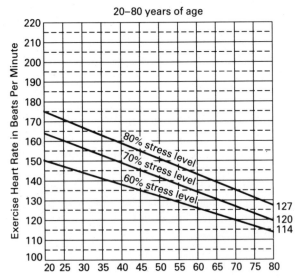

20–80 years of age

Table 2.1

**Ten-Second Exercise Heart Rate
Converted to Beats Per Minute**

10-Second Exercise Heart Rate	1-Minute Conversion
15	90
16	96
17	102
18	108
19	114
20	120
21	126
22	132
23	138
24	144
25	150
26	156
27	162
28	168
29	174
30	180

Table 2.2

**Ten-Second Exercise Heart Rate
For Age Ranges From 15 to 89**

	10-Second Exercise Heart Rate		
Age	Lower Limit		Upper Limit
6–10	24	—	29
11–19	25	—	30
20–29	24	—	28
30–39	22	—	27
40–49	21	—	25
50–59	20	—	24
60–69	19	—	22
70–79	18	—	21
80–89	16	—	19

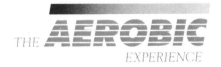
THE **AEROBIC**
EXPERIENCE

Once you have become familiar with the skills presented in this book, you will want to create routines that allow you to exercise at an intensity level that gives you a training effect. In Chapters 4 and 5, you will see routine charts like the one below, for you to complete using appropriate skills.

Seq refers to the sequence of the music, i.e., introduction, phrase, chorus, interlude, etc.

Reps refers to the number of times a particular skill or movement will be repeated within the sequence.

Skill identifies the specific skill variation or combination to be performed.

Music count refers to the number of music counts needed to perform the sequence.

Routine Chart

Seq	Reps	Skills	Music Count

Warm-Up and Cool-Down Exercises

The first part of every aerobic dance workout should consist of warm-up exercises to increase circulation and gently stretch and strengthen each muscle group. In this phase of the workout, you are "gearing up"—not going at full speed yet; so you will want to choose music that is invigorating but not pushing—music that motivates you to move but doesn't make you want to jump around quite yet.

The exercises illustrated in this chapter, in the sequence they appear, constitute a safe and enjoyable warm-up routine, and they may be used for cooling down after a workout. These exercises are described in Tables 3.1, 3.2, and 3.3. Table 3.1 presents a series of relaxed movements of the arms and legs performed to increase the blood flow to all parts of the body. Tables 3.2 and 3.3 present stretching and strengthening exercises for specific muscle groups.

Referring to the tables, you will see that the first column (Tables 3.2 and 3.3) names the exercise and identifies the muscle group being conditioned. The second column in Tables 3.1 through 3.3 describes each exercise at the medium level. Pay attention to the precautions. Figures depicting the exercise at the medium level are also cited. The figures, when necessary, show the most common errors made in performing the exercise so that you can correct yourself. The final column explains how the exercise can be modified for the high-level and the low-level participant.

Here are two general rules to follow when engaging in exercise:

1. Do not bob or bounce on a stretched muscle. Sustained, controlled stretching will prepare the body for aerobic activity more effectively, increase flexibility, and minimize the possibility of straining or tearing the muscle tissue.

Table 3.1   Circulation Exercises

Figures	Medium Level	Variations for Low and **High** Levels
Figure 3.1	Step from one foot to the other, pushing weight from toes to ball of foot along outer border to heel. Swing arms from side to side at various levels.	**Low**: Hold support for balance.
Figure 3.2	Continue treading with feet as you extend arms and hands upward and outward.	**High**: Increase intensity of foot tread and elbow circles.
Figure 3.3	Continue stepping with feet as you rotate elbows in circular movement.	
Figure 3.4	Step and touch or swing foot forward and move arms in various patterns (see Chapter 4, "Arm Movements").	
Figure 3.5	Extend arms sideward with elbows slightly bent. Circle with backward turning motion; repeat forward. **Precaution**: Keep elbows bent to avoid shoulder-joint trauma.	**Low**: Circle one arm at a time if necessary. **High**: Increase size of circle.

AEROBIC DANCE

2. Follow correct principles of body alignment when performing each exercise. Avoid movements that result in pressure at an angle to the weight-bearing surface. For example, when performing jumping jacks, if you land with your feet farther apart than shoulder width, you place undue stress at the ankle and knee joints.

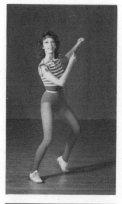

Figure 3.1
Foot Tread and Arm Swing

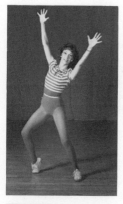

Figure 3.2
Foot Tread and Arm Extension

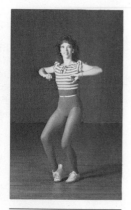

Figure 3.3
Foot Tread and Elbow Extension

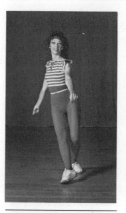

Figure 3.4
Toe Touch Forward

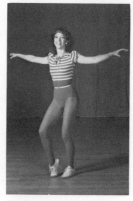

Figure 3.5
Arm Rotation and Foot Tread

Warm-Up and Cool-Down Exercises

Table 3.2 Sustained Stretching Exercises

Exercise and Muscle Group	Medium Level	Variations for **Low** and **High** Levels
Lateral stretch: upper torso Figure 3.6	With a slow, continuous movement, push right arm high overhead, bending upper body slightly toward left. Repeat with left hand high.	
Figure 3.7	**Precaution:** Keep the knees bent and both heels on the floor. Do not pulse, bounce, or bob. Do not allow knees to roll inward. Keep knees directly over feet.	
Shoulder-girdle stretch Figure 3.8	Reach the right arm up and over the right shoulder and the left arm under the left shoulder. Try to clasp your palms together in the center of your back	
Neck stretch: neck and shoulders Figure 3.9	Slowly roll head sideward, bringing right ear toward right shoulder; repeat to left.	**Low:** Hold to support for balance. **High:** Gently pull head with opposite hand.
Figure 3.10	**Precaution:** Do not roll your head backward beyond the perpendicular line with your shoulders.	
Toe tapper: tibialis anterior (front of lower leg) and posterior (back of lower leg) Figure 3.11	In a standing position or leaning against a wall with weight supported on heels, tap your toes to the floor.	**Low:** Tap one foot at a time or tap both feet while seated. Figure 3.12

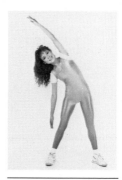

Figure 3.6
Lateral Stretch

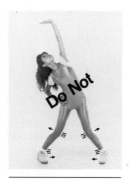

Figure 3.7
Precaution: Ankle
and Knee Trauma

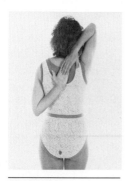

Figure 3.8
Shoulder-Girdle
Stretch

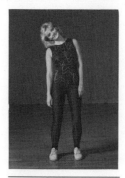

Figure 3.9
Neck Stretch

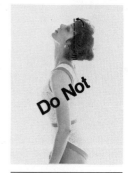

Figure 3.10
Precaution: Tension
on Vertebrae

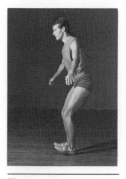

Figure 3.11
Toe Tapper

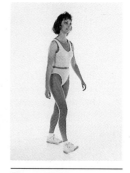

Figure 3.12
Toe Tapper, Low Level

Warm-Up and Cool-Down Exercises

Table 3.2 (continued)

Exercise and Muscle Group	Medium Level	Variations for **Low** and **High** Levels
Torso stretch: upper torso Figure 3.13	Stand with feet in shoulder-width position and knees flexed. Stretch arms alternately (1) both up, (2) right arm to right side, (3) left arm to left side, (4) both arms forward. **Precaution:** Keep movement smooth. Eliminate ballistic movement.	**Low:** One arm at a time. If necessary, perform while seated on a straight-back chair. **High:** Increase intensity of stretch.
Wide-stride plié and lateral stretch: inner thighs, upper torso Figure 3.14	In wide-stride position (feet in 2nd position), bend knees over feet. Contract abdominal muscles. Hold position while stretching upward alternately, left and right. **Precaution:** Perform with your knees directly in line with your feet to avoid pressure at the knee and ankle joints.	**Low:** Bend knees only as far as you can while maintaining knees directly over feet. (Hold to support for balance.) **High:** Bend knees deeper; extend torso stretch.
Wide-stride plié with heel lifts: inner thighs, muscles of calf, and foot Figure 3.15	In wide-stride position (1) raise heels up (maintain weight on balls of feet), (2) lower heels to floor, (3) move arms up and down with heel motion.	**Low:** Minimize knee bend. Maintain knees over feet. (Hold to support for balance.) **High:** Bend knees deeper. Extend ankle, stretch through torso.
Tug-of-war: upper back Figure 3.16	Round back; contract muscles of abdomen, hips, buttocks, arms, and shoulders. Keep knees bent.	**Low:** Hold to support, to maintain balance, or perform while seated on a straight-back chair. **High:** Increase effort.

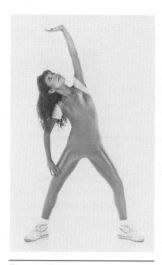

Figure 3.13
Torso Stretch

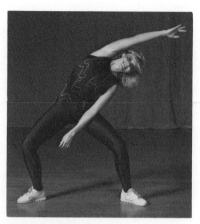

Figure 3.14
Wide-Stride Plié and
Lateral Stretch

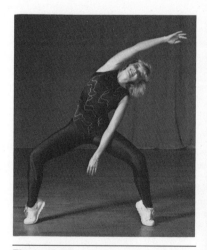

Figure 3.15
Wide-Stride Plié and Lateral
Stretch with Heel Lifts

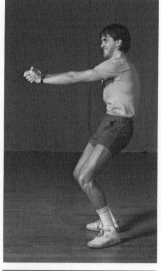

Figure 3.16
Tug-of-War

Warm-Up and Cool-Down Exercises

Table 3.2 (continued)

Exercise and Muscle Group	Medium Level	Variations for **Low** and **High** Levels
Back hand-clasp: upper back, chest Figure 3.17	In standing position with knees bent, clasp hands behind back and raise as far forward as possible. **Precaution**: Keep head in line with shoulders.	**Low**: Stand with side against wall to maintain balance. Keep your head and shoulders above the level of your heart. **High**: Move arms high and forward over back, and bend forward to touch chest to thighs.
Hamstring stretch: hamstring (back of thighs and buttocks) Figure 3.18 Figure 3.19	From a crouched position with knees bent, rib cage on thighs, hands holding heels, gently straighten knees maintaining rib cage on thighs.	**Low**: Perform the "nose to knees" exercise while seated on floor. **High**: Forcefully hold (glue) chest to thighs. Place nose to right knee. Repeat to left. Place head between knees.
Tailor sit lift: inner thighs Figure 3.20	Sitting with soles of feet together, hands next to buttocks, lift seat off floor and roll pelvic girdle under, push knees outward and downward.	**Low**: Gentle sustained movement. **High**: Forceful but continuous sustained movement.
Sitting wide stride: hips, back, thighs Figure 3.21 Figure 3.22 Figure 3.23	Maintaining the above leg position, gently extend legs out into a sitting stride, body forward, chest toward floor. Lateral stretch can also be performed in this position. **Precaution**: Roll the knees outward, keeping the knee in line with your turned-out feet.	

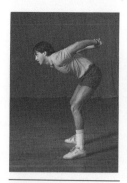

**Figure 3.17
Back Hand Clasp**

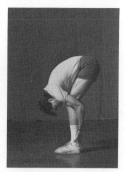

**Figure 3.18
Hamstring Stretch**

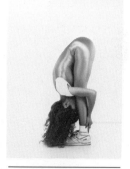

**Figure 3.19
Hamstring Stretch,
High Level**

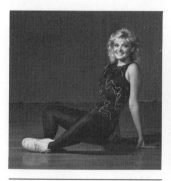

**Figure 3.20
Tailor Sit Lift**

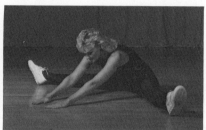

**Figure 3.21
Sitting Wide Stride**

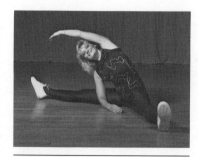

**Figure 3.22
Sitting Wide Stride and
Lateral Stretch**

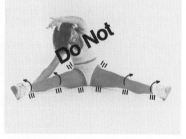

**Figure 3.23
Precaution: Hip, Knee, and
Ankle Trauma**

Warm-Up and Cool-Down Exercises

Table 3.2 (continued)

Exercise and Muscle Group	Medium Level	Variations for **Low** and **High** Levels
Lower back stretch: muscle in lower-back Figure 3.24	Lie on back, left leg extended, right leg bent. Clasp hands around right knee; slowly pull to right shoulder. Repeat with opposite leg.	**High:** Increase the stretch by pulling both knees toward your shoulders with a slow sustained stretch. Figure 3.25
Nose to knees: hamstrings, buttocks, back Figure 3.26	In a sitting position with knees bent, rib cage on thighs, nose on knees; gently extend legs. Maintain rib-cage-on-thighs position.	**Low:** Straighten legs so far as you can maintain chest-on-thigh position. **High:** Flex ankles while pushing legs forward. Keep chest "glued" to thighs.
Hip flexor, quad stretch: muscles on front of thigh and down front of lower leg Figure 3.27 Figure 3.28	While in a side-lying position with bottom leg bent for support, bend the top leg (keep foot and lower leg in line with your thigh). Grasp top of foot and pull while pushing the upper leg back against the forward force stretching the thigh muscles. Repeat several times for a sustained stretch on each thigh. **Precaution:** Maintain a space between the calf (gastrocnemius) and the back of the thigh (hamstrings) to avoid pressure on the knee joint. Do not arch your back; keep the stretch in the quadricep muscle.	

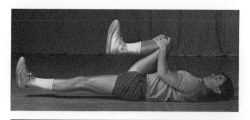

Figure 3.24
Lower Back Stretch

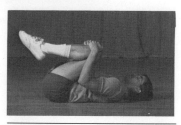

Figure 3.25
Lower Back Stretch, High Level

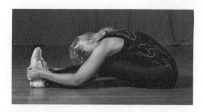

Figure 3.26
Nose to Knees, Hamstring
Stretch

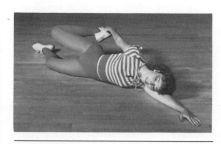

Figure 3.27
Quadriceps Stretch

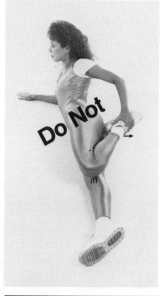

Figure 3.28
Precaution: Lower Back and
Knee Joint Trauma

Table 3.2 (continued)

Exercise and Muscle Group	Medium Level	Variations for **Low** and **High** Levels
Treadmill: ankle and heel cord Figure 3.29	With weight on hands and balls of feet in an inverted **V**-position, tread slowly, right foot then left foot, pushing heel toward floor. This exercise can also be performed in an upright position with hands against a wall or stable support.	**Low:** While holding a forward leaning position against a wall or stable support, alternately tread feet, pushing heel toward the floor. Figure 3.30 **High:** Extend the inverted **V**-position for greater treading action.
Four position leg-and-hip exercise: inside of thigh Figure 3.31	a. Assume a wide-spread squat position with hands cupped over knee cap. Move slowly to right side for a sustained stretch of inside of thigh. Repeat to left.	**Low:** forward lunge position; hold on to chair or stable support if needed. Figure 3.32
Quadriceps, posterior, thigh Figure 3.33	b. Assume a forward-lean position, keeping heel of 90° bent leg on floor; lower hips toward floor. Repeat with opposite leg forward.	**Low:** Standing in a forward-stride position, lean over bent front leg. Figure 3.34

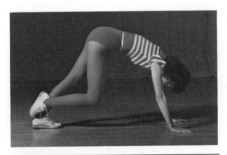

Figure 3.29
Treadmill

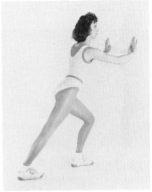

Figure 3.30
Treadmill, Low Level

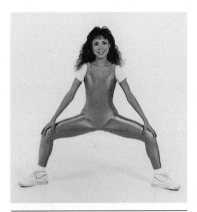

**Figure 3.31
Four Position Leg and Hip
Exercise (position a)**

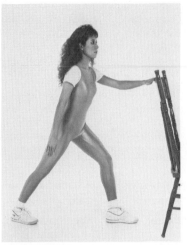

**Figure 3.32
Four Position Forward Lunge,
Low Level**

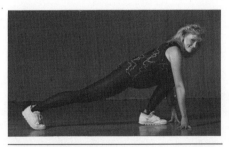

**Figure 3.33
Four Position Leg and Hip Exercise
(position b)**

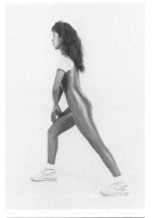

**Figure 3.34
Four Position Leg and
Hip Exercise, Low Level
(position b)**

Table 3.2 (continued)

Exercise and Muscle Group	Medium Level	Variations for **Low** and **High** Levels
Quadriceps, hip flexor, gastrocnemius, soleus, achilles Figure 3.35	c. Assume a forward-lean position, keeping hips in line with shoulders, forward leg bent at knee with 60° heel pushing toward floor.	**Low:** Standing in a forward-stride position, push forward over bent front leg. Figure 3.36
Hamstring, buttock, achilles Figure 3.37	d. Assuming a forward-stride position, keeping knees softly bent, lean upper torso over front leg.	**Low:** Standing with legs in forward-stride position, bend upper body forward. Figure 3.38
Figure 3.39	e. Extend the stretch by lifting the toe of the forward foot.	**High:** Extend stride; raise toe of front leg.
Pretzel: lower back and buttock Figure 3.40	While seated in position (a) or (b), pull one knee toward shoulders. Hold for a sustained stretch.	**High:** Increase pull toward shoulder. Figure 3.41

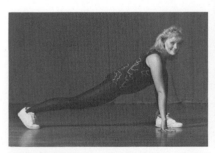

Figure 3.35
Four Position Leg and Hip Exercise (position c)

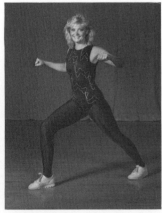

Figure 3.36
Four Position Leg and Hip Exercise, Low Level

AEROBIC DANCE

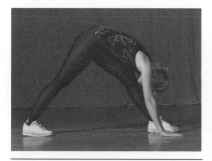

Figure 3.37
Four Position Leg and Hip
Exercise (position d)

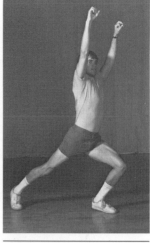

Figure 3.38
Four Position Leg and Hip
Exercise, Low Level
(position d)

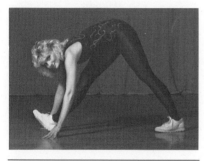

Figure 3.39
Four Position Leg and Hip
Exercise (position e)

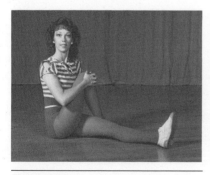

Figure 3.40
Pretzel, Medium Level

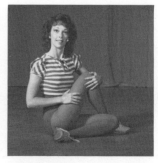

Figure 3.41
Pretzel, High Level

Warm-Up and Cool-Down Exercises

Table 3.3 Strengthening Exercises

Exercise and Muscle Group	Medium Level	Variations for **Low** and **High** Levels
Abdominal curls: abdominal muscle group Figure 3.42	From a starting position of sitting with shoulders in line with the hip joint, back rounded in a C position and abdominal muscles contracted tightly, move your body slowly, rolling down each vertebrae to touch your upper back to floor; return to starting position. Maintain C position throughout the exercise.	**Low:** (a) Use hands to assist rolling up and down by pulling on backs of thighs or (b) reach arms toward knees. Maintain C position throughout. Figure 3.43 Figure 3.44 **High:** Move as slowly as possible, keeping muscles contracted with feet flat on floor and arms pressed tight to rib cage. Figure 3.45
Push ups: arms and shoulders Figure 3.46	Assume one of the three pictured positions. By bending your elbows, lower your body to touch your chest to the floor. Perform as many as you can at your highest level.	**Low** Figure 3.47 **High** Figure 3.48

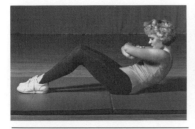

Figure 3.42
Abdominal Curl, Medium Level

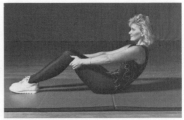

Figure 3.43
Abdominal Curl, Low Level (a)

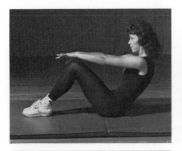

Figure 3.44
Abdominal Curl, Low level
(b)

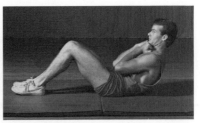

Figure 3.45
Abdominal Curl, High Level

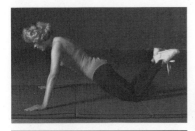

Figure 3.46
Pushups, Medium Level

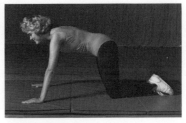

Figure 3.47
Pushups, Low Level

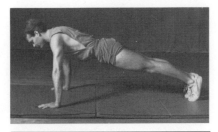

Figure 3.48
Pushups, High Level

Table 3.3 (continued)

Exercise and Muscle Group	Medium Level	Variations for **Low** and **High** Levels
Figure 3.49	**Precaution**: Maintain a straight line from shoulder to knees or feet to avoid undue strain on the vertebrae of your lower back. Do not let your lower back sag when performing pushups or other horizontal body movements.	Figure 3.50

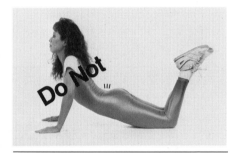

Figure 3.49
Precaution: Lower Back Trauma

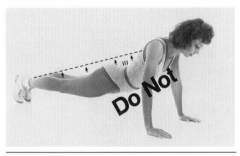

Figure 3.50
Precaution: Lower Back Trauma

AEROBIC DANCE

Arm Movements

Arm movements are performed for several reasons. They vary the intensity of the workout, increase the flexibility and strength of the arm and shoulder-girdle muscles, increase the neuromuscular coordination of arms and legs, and give style and beauty to the skill being performed.

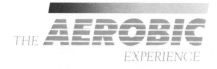
THE **AEROBIC** EXPERIENCE

Practice the arm movements shown in Figures 4.1 through 4.20. Sit or stand with body in good postural alignment. When the movement becomes easy to perform, add a walking or running step in coordination with the arm movements. Practice a variety of steps and arm movements with selected musical accompaniment.

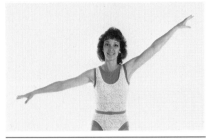

Figure 4.1 Airplane Arms Extend both arms in a diagonal. Move arms up and down without breaking diagonal.

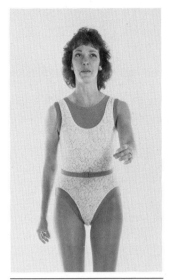

Figure 4.2 Alternate Arm Swings Swing arms freely, one arm moving forward high, the other downward and back.

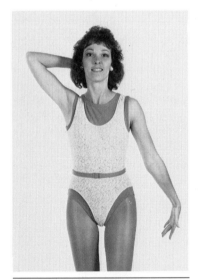

Figure 4.3 Back Slapper Extend one arm forward in front of body. At the same time, reach the other arm over the shoulder, slapping back of shoulder blade. Alternate left and right.

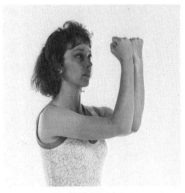

Figure 4.4 Bent-Arm Press To start, raise arms shoulder height—elbows at 90 degrees and palms turned to center. Press arms forward and touch together in front of chest.

AEROBIC DANCE

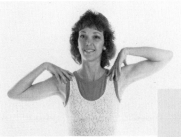

Figure 4.5 Chicken Wings Elbows bent with arms at side of body, hands on shoulders, move arms in flapping fashion.

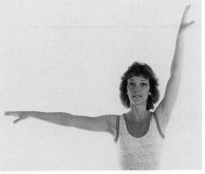

Figure 4.6 L Arms Extend right arm, sidewards, left arm high overhead. On count 1, bring both arms down to slap sides of thighs. Alternate arm positions.

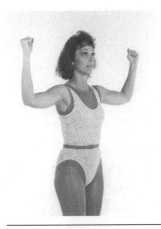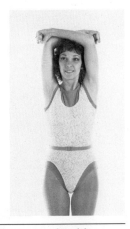

Figure 4.7 Macho Arms Raise arms shoulder high, elbows bent at a 90-degree angle, fists clenched. On count 1, press arms together in front of chest. (2) On count 2, bring arms overhead to form a square.

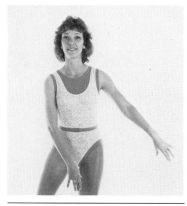

Figure 4.8 Pendulum Arms
Swing arms from side to side in front of body.

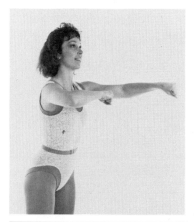

Figure 4.9 Punching Make a fist and alternately extend arms forward in front of shoulders.

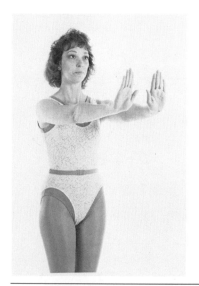

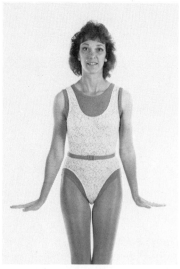

Figure 4.10 Push Arms Extend arms out from chest, wrists flexed, palms forward.   a. front b. down

AEROBIC DANCE

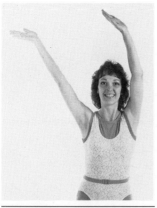

Figure 4.11 Rainbow Arms
Bring arms high overhead
and swing in an arc from
right to left.

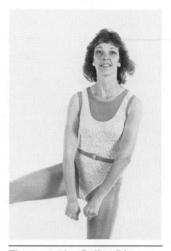

Figure 4.12 Sailor Dig
With both hands held low in
front of body, on count 1,
bend elbows outward and
bring hands to waist height.
On count 2, forcefully
extend in a washboard
scrubbing action. Single
Dig: Using same action,
bend right elbow as you
extend left elbow.

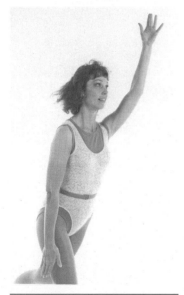

Figure 4.13 Scissor Arms
Arms are straight in front of
body: One above head, the
other down by side. Alternate
positions.

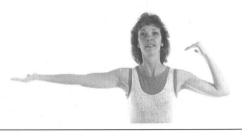

Figure 4.14 Shoulder Touch Extend one arm to side with other arm bent at elbow and hand touching shoulder. Alternate from bent to extended, right and left. Variations: 1. With hands touching shoulders and elbows shoulder high in front, extend arms forward and then back to shoulder touch position. 2. Alternate right and left arm, forward and back.

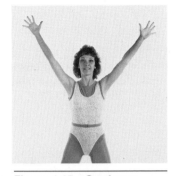

Figure 4.15 Starburst Arms burst up and out from shoulders overhead; fingers are spread.

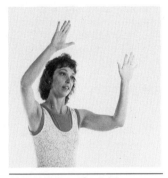

Figure 4.16 Sunshine Arms Starting with hands in front of shoulders (elbows bent), extend both arms up with light bouncy movements. Take fingers from closed to open position on each count.

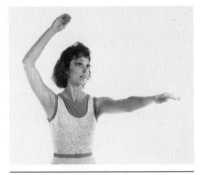

Figure 4.17 Swim Arms Hands in front of chest, alternately extend arms up and overhead and out to sides in a front crawl swimming stroke.

AEROBIC DANCE

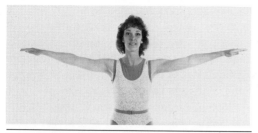

Figure 4.18 T Arms Starting with arms down touching sides of thighs, raise to shoulder level and return to sides of thighs.

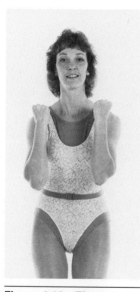

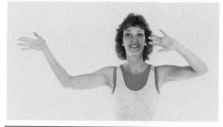

Figure 4.20 Windshield Wipers Hands are in front of chest, fingers spread, and elbows extended sideward shoulder high. Move forearms and hands in and out sideward.
a. both arms in and out
b. arms alternated, in then out

Figure 4.19 Throw Catch Bend arms with hands in front of shoulders. Throw arms out then bend them in. Variation: Repeat same action down in front of thighs.

CHOREOGRAPHING YOUR OWN ROUTINES

Now you are ready to create your own routines using the arm movements and the soft-rebound and smooth-impact skills as illustrated in Chapters 5 and 6. Start at the low-skill and intensity level and progress gradually to the intermediate and high levels as you increase in fitness and skill. Each simple routine includes skills that you can perform easily as well as some more complex moves. If a skill is difficult for you, substitute a skill with which you are more comfortable. We begin with routines that use smooth-impact skills then show routines that use soft-rebound moves, but you should vary the two types of skills according to your own needs and preferences.

The following steps will help you get started:

1. Select music with a good steady beat. Study the music and count the beats relative to introduction, phrase, chorus, interlude, etc.
2. Select three or four skills that are easy for you to perform.
3. Practice walking or running in place with the music accompaniment. Walking or running can be used as a transition movement between skills.
4. You are now ready to sequence your skills and transition movements with the music and "chart" the routine.

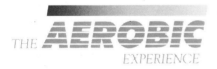

THE **AEROBIC** EXPERIENCE

Aerobic routines can be charted using only one locomotor skill and a series of arm movements.

SOFT-REBOUND ROUTINE

Selected skills: run in place, run w/high knees, run w/seat kicker. Arms: alternate swing, sunshine, bent arms press, back slapper, chicken wings.

Select music that has a good 4/4 beat and a tempo appropriate for your personal training zone.

The example in Table 4.1 charts a routine to music that has a 16-count introduction and 16 phrases of 32 counts each.

Table 4.1   Soft-Rebound Routine

Seq	Reps	Skills	Music Count
Intro	16	Run in place Arms: alternate swings	16
I	32	Run in place Arms: sunshine	32
II	32	Run in place lifting knees up and forward on each step Arms: Bent-arm press	32
III	32	Run in place lifting feet up and backward on each step (seat kicker) Arms: back slapper	32
IV	32	Run in place Arms: chicken wings	32
I, II, III, IV	128	Repeat 3×	384

Smooth-Impact Skills

This chapter describes smooth-impact routines. Photographs (Figures 5.1 through 5.28) are used to illustrate the skills listed for these routines. Practice each of the skills illustrated before doing the sequences charted in the sample smooth-impact routines.

Performing Variations for High and Low Levels

High level is achieved by bending the knees deeper, extending the body into each movement, and moving the arms vigorously. *Low level* is achieved by performing each movement with the knees slightly bent and the arms moving rhythmically and close to the body.

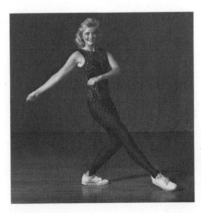

Figure 5.1 Front Basic Step on left foot and extend right foot diagonally forward. Repeat to right. Swing arms rhythmically.

AEROBIC DANCE

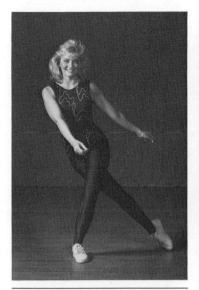

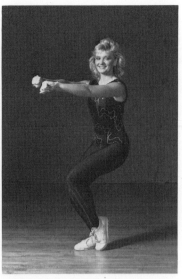

Figure 5.2 Back Basic Step right on right foot. Extend left leg diagonally behind and touch ball of foot to floor. Repeat to left.

Figure 5.3 Side Basic Assuming illustrated position, step right foot sideward right. At same time, swing arms outward shoulder height. On count 2, touch left foot to right foot, bringing arms together in front of body. Repeat to left.

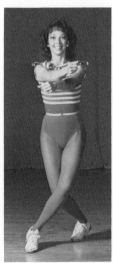

Figure 5.4 Grapevine Open Perform a sequence: Step right, cross behind with left, step right. On count 4, lift left leg high diagonally forward. Repeat same sequence to left.

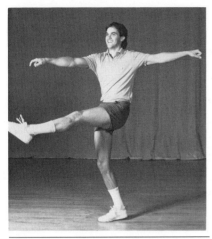

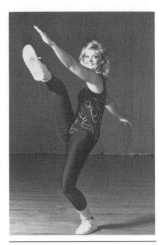

Figure 5.5   Step Kick-Front   Step left, sinking into movement by bending knees. Kick right leg forward and touch left hand to right foot. Repeat right.

Figure 5.6   Step Kick-Front, High Level

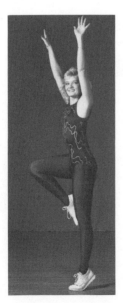

Figure 5.7 Schottische   Step 3 times, moving forward. Hop on count 4 (lift body high, maintaining contact with floor on ball of foot); lift bent leg high in the air. Repeat, starting on opposite foot.

AEROBIC DANCE

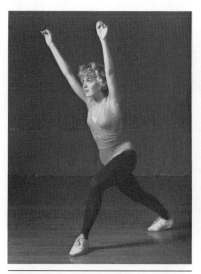

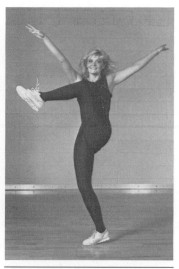

Figure 5.8 Deep Lunge With weight on left foot, knee bent at 90-degree angle, right leg back, and a sustained stretch, push heel to floor. Raise arms high over shoulders. Repeat to right by making half turn as you place weight on right foot and extend left leg back for heel-cord stretch.

Figure 5.9 Step with Knee Lift Step left. Raise right knee as high as you can. Move arms sideward. Repeat on opposite foot.

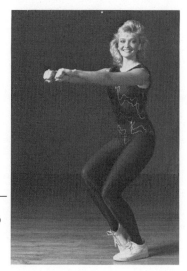

Figure 5.10 Chassé Do continuous (4) side-basic steps to the right. Repeat to left. Maintain "sit" position throughout the sequence.

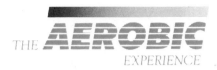

SMOOTH-IMPACT ROUTINE

Selected skills: Front basic, side basic, grapevine open, step kick.

The music selected for this routine has a 12-count introduction, 9 phrases of 32 counts each, an interlude of 32 counts, and 5 more phrases of 32 counts each.

The sample routine chart using the skills and music described is completed as shown here. (Adjust the chart to coincide with your music selection.)

Seq	Reps	Skills	Music Count
Intro	6	Step/heel touch	12
I	4	Front basic	8
	4	Back basic	8
	8	Side basic	16
II	4	Grapevine open	16
III	8	Side basic	16
	4	Grapevine open	16
IV	4	Front basic	16
	4	Side basic	16
	4	Back basic	16
	4	Side basic	16
	4	Grapevine open	16
I		Repeat I	32
II		Repeat II 2 ×	32
III		Repeat III	32
II		Repeat II 2 ×	32

Interlude	4	Step kick front (four in each direction: forward, side right, back, side left)	32
I, II, III, IV		Repeat to end of music	

Now that you have learned the basic steps, you can choreograph new routines. Simply change the music and add one or two new skills.

Routine 5.1

Suggested Music: "Body 10"
Style: Smooth Impact
Choreographer: Claudia Hill

		Skills	Music	Skill Variations	
Seq	Reps	Medium Level	Count	High Level	Low Level
Intro	16	Light jog	16		
I	8	Side basic	16	Increase knee bend; extend body into each movement. Use vigorous arm movements	Relaxed knees
	8	Front basic	16		Small side step; relaxed arm movements
	8	Back basic	16		
	8	Side basic	16		
II	4	Schottische F, B, F, B	16	Lift knee high on count 4	Relaxed movement
	4	Grapevine R, L, R, L	16	Leg lift on count 4	Hesitation touch on count 4
III	16	Lunge step (4–2–1)	32	Use deep-knee lunge; vigorous arm movements	Relaxed knees and relaxed arm movements

Routine 5.1 (continued)

Seq	Reps	Skills Medium Level	Music Count	Skill Variations High Level	Low Level
I	8 8	Side basic Front basic	16 16		
II		Repeat			
III		Repeat			
IV	4	Turning basic	16	Travel with turn	Side basic, omit turn
	4	Turning basic w/windmill arms	16	Extend arms and move in large circle	Side basic, omit turn
I	8 8	Side basic Front basic	16 16		
II		Repeat			
IV		Repeat			
III		Repeat			
I		Side Basic	16		

Routine 5.2

Suggested Music: "Up-N-At-Em"
Style: Smooth Impact
Choreographer: Bard Hill

Seq	Reps	Skills Medium Level	Music Count	Skill Variations High Level	Low Level
Intro a	8	Side basic	16	Bend knees throughout.	Easy up/down movement with knees.
b	4	Grapevine (R–L–R–L)	16	Lift leg on count 4	Touch on count 4

AEROBIC DANCE

Seq	Reps	Skills Medium Level	Music Count	Skill Variations High Level	Low Level
I	8	Front basic	16	Extend side step	Small side step
	8	Back basic	16	Extend side step	Small side step
		Repeat	32		
II	4	Side basic	8	Extend body into each move; bend knees more deeply	
	4	Front basic	8		
	4	Side basic	8		
	4	Back basic	8		
III	1	Grapevine to right	4	Kick above waist level	Step touch front
	2	Step kick	4		
		Repeat 3 ×'s (L–R–L)	24		
Intro b	4	Grapevine (R–L–R–L)	16		
I			32		
III			32		
IV	16	Knee lift (elbow to knee)	32	High knee lift	Lift knee slightly
Interlude	16	Chassé	32	Travel front and back	Perform in place.
	16	Step and kick	32	High side kick	Cross touch side.
Intro b	4	Grapevine (R–L–R–L)	16		
I			32		
II			32		
III			32		
IV			32		

MORE SMOOTH-IMPACT SKILLS

Figures 5.11 through 5.28 show a number of other smooth-impact skills which you can substitute in any of the three previous routines or use to make your own.

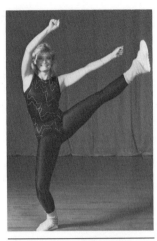

Figure 5.11   Step Kick-Sideward   Step right. Raise left leg sideward. Use arms to maintain balance.

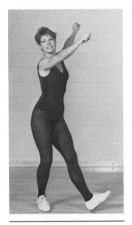

Figure 5.12   Freddie Step on right foot. Extend left leg forward and touch heel to floor. Swing arms upward. Repeat, starting with left foot.

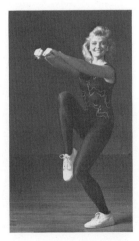

Figure 5.13   Butterfly Wings (1) Step on right foot; at same time touch left knee to chest and bring arms together in front of shoulders. (2) Step on left foot; at same time tuck right knee to chest and open arms to **T** position. Sink into each step by bending knees.

AEROBIC DANCE

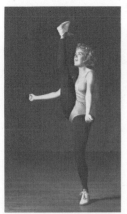

Figure 5.14 Chorus Line Kick (1) Step right; at same time lift left knee to chest; (2) touch left foot to floor and swing it immediately into a high kick. Repeat on opposite foot. Repeat entire sequence.

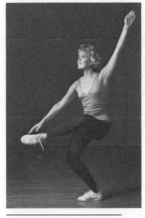

Figure 5.16 Jester Run Step left. Raise right foot in front. Reach left hand forward to touch right foot (sink into each step). Repeat to right.

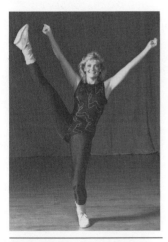

Figure 5.15 Open Basic Step to left on left foot. Open arms wide above shoulders and lift right leg sideward. Repeat to right.

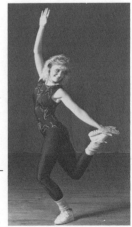

Figure 5.17 Hop Scotch Hop on right foot. Lift left foot diagonally backward. Touch left foot with right hand as you hop on right foot. Repeat by starting on left foot.

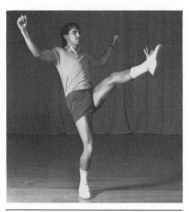

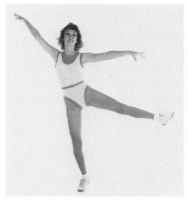

Figure 5.18 Rocking Horse
(1) Rock forward with weight on right leg; (2) rock backward, putting weight on left leg. Repeat this rocking action several times. Repeat with opposite leg forward.

Figure 5.19 Fly Away With weight on right leg, raise left leg up and down sideward left. Raise left hand diagonally up and down in rhythm with leg. Repeat this action 1 to 4 times, changing weight to left leg, and repeat action 1 to 4 times, raising right leg and arm.

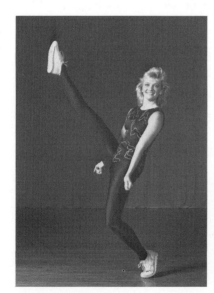

Figure 5.20 Progressive Step Touch Lift On count one, step on right foot. On count two, extend left leg forward and touch floor with foot. On count three, lift that same foot high forward. Repeat by stepping on left foot.

AEROBIC DANCE

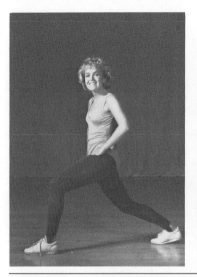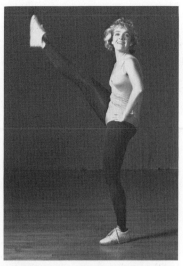

Figure 5.21 Jazz Kick/Achilles Stretch On count 1, step backward with right foot, stretch the Achilles tendon, and bring that same foot into a high kick. Return to standing position. Repeat with left foot.

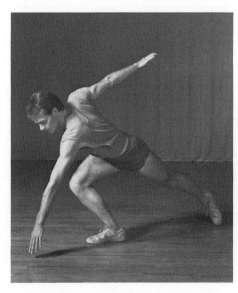

Figure 5.22 Charleston
A four-count sequence:
(1) Step forward on right foot; (2) swing left leg high, swing right arm to left foot; (3) step back on left foot; (4) extend right leg backward, lean forward, and touch hand to floor. Repeat 4 to 8 times. Reverse pattern by stepping forward on left foot, etc.

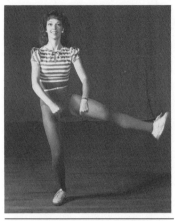

Figure 5.23   Cowboy Kicks
Kick right leg high. Raise arms
alternately high and low in
front of body. Repeat with left
leg.

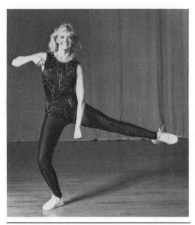

Figure 5.24   Pendulum
Pendulum action moves sideward.
Step left. Raise right leg sideward,
hands digging forward. Repeat
right with quick weight change.

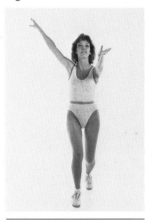

Figure 5.25   Pivot Basic
In a forward stride
position, swing arms up
in air and pivot both feet
one-half turn (180
degrees). Lean forward
into new direction.
Repeat and turn back to
original position.

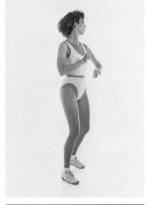

Figure 5.26   Pivot Turn
In a forward stride
position, plant the
forward foot. Make one-
half turn (180 degrees) by
stepping back foot
forward and pivoting
both feet in place. Step
forward in the new
direction and repeat the
entire sequence.

AEROBIC DANCE

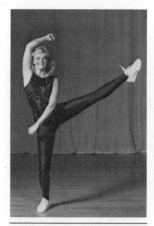

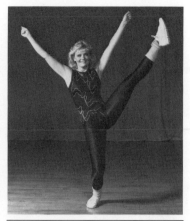

Figure 5.27   Cross Step with Side Kick   Cross left foot diagonally forward. Swing right leg sideward right. Cross right foot diagonally forward. Swing left leg sideward left.

Figure 5.28   Sunburst   Step left on left foot. Lift right foot high right, and swing arms high in air. Repeat stepping right on right foot and lifting left foot high.

Soft-Rebound Skills

When performing the soft-rebound moves, you must practice landing softly. Think about not hearing your feet hit the floor. The energy expended should be in the direction of the takeoff, and the soft landing is achieved by a cushioning effect as a result of bending at each of the joints of the body.

Performing these skills requires an excessive number of takeoffs and landings during each aerobic workout session. Consequently, there is a relatively high probability that stress and strain will result. Preventative measures, such as appropriate cushion-soled shoes, resilient surfaces, proper warm-up to increase circulation and to stretch and strengthen muscles should precede aerobic participation.

To vary the intensity of soft-rebound skills for the low level, keep one foot in contact with the floor and move arms rhythmically and close to your body. Low level is commensurate to walking.

For the medium level, feet can be off the floor at the same time; but leg lifts or kicks should not be higher than hip level. The arms move rhythmically and as high as shoulder level. Medium level is commensurate to jogging.

For the high-intensity level, legs are kicked shoulder high, arms move vigorously, and both feet are often off the floor. High intensity is commensurate to running.

Photos accompany the description of each skill presented in Tables 6.1 and 6.2. The skills are shown progressively, from the simple to the more complex. If a skill is difficult for you, practice it before the aerobic workout session. After difficult skills are learned, they should be included in the Skill Review Phase of each aerobic workout session until they become a part of your skill repertoire. When you are familiar with the skills, perform the simple routine or a routine you choreograph yourself that includes these skills.

Table 6.2 shows various other soft-rebound skills and variations. Following this table are still other soft-rebound routines. You can use the skills to substitute in any of the previous routines or to make your own routines.

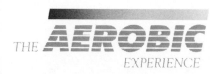

THE AEROBIC EXPERIENCE

SOFT-REBOUND ROUTINE

Selected skills: Heel touch, cowboy kicks, twosies, and pendulum

The music chosen for this routine has a 16-count introduction and 20 phrases of 32 counts each. The following chart includes skills listed in Table 6.1. (Adjust the repetitions on the chart to coincide with your musical selection.)

Seq	Reps	Skills	Music Count
Intro	16	Step 3, hop in place/sunshine hands	16
I	4	Heel touch, alternate right and left	8
	8	Run in place	8
		Repeat	16
II	4	Cowboy kicks, alternate right and left	8
	8	Run in place	8
		Repeat	16
III	4	Twosies	8
	8	Run in place	8
		Repeat	16
IV	8	Pendulum	8
	8	Run in place	8
		Repeat sequences I, II, III, and IV four more times to end of music.	16

Table 6.1   Soft-Rebound Skills

Skills

Heel touch
  Rebound from left foot to right, and at same time touch left heel to floor in front.

Repeat with rebound to left foot, and touch right heel to floor.

Figure 6.1

Cowboy kicks
  Step-hop on right leg. At same time, kick left leg high in air, bending at knee and ankle.

Figure 6.2

Twosies
  Hop twice on right leg, swing left leg sideward, hop twice on left leg, swing right leg sideward. Swing arms alternately high and low with leg action.

Figure 6.3

Pendulum swing
  While making a quick change of weight from right foot to left, swing lower body sideward right.

Repeat action while making quick transfer to right foot.

Figure 6.4

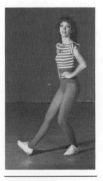 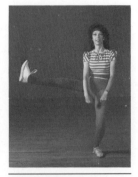

Figure 6.1
Heel Touch

Figure 6.2
Cowboy Kicks

AEROBIC DANCE

	Variations	
High Level	Low Level	Safety Precautions
Increase height of re-bound, alternately swing arms high overhead.	Step on right foot and touch left heel to floor in front of body. Repeat left.	Touch heel lightly to floor to avoid bruising. Hold to support for balance.
Perform with high leg kick diagonally forward.	Step right, kick left leg diagonally forward, repeat left.	
Increase arm swings, crossing in front of body. Increase leg swing, swing sideward.	Step left and swing right leg sideward right. Step right and swing left leg side-ward left.	Hold to support to maintain balance, if necessary.
With arms moving up and down in sailor dig action, move your lower body vigorously at hips, lifting legs high, alternately left and right.	Step right, lift left leg sideward; repeat left. Progress to smooth running action, mov-ing opposite foot side-ward on each step.	Warm up carefully with low back, hip, buttocks, and thigh exercises.

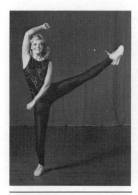

Figure 6.3
Twosies

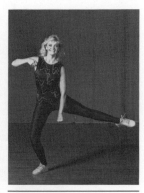

Figure 6.4
Pendulum Swing

Table 6.1   Soft-Rebound Skills Continued

Skills

Hop with knee lift
While hopping on left foot, touch right foot to floor, then lift right knee high in air.

Repeat with left foot while hopping right.

Figure 6.5

Fly-Away
Starting position: Hands on sides, weight centered on both feet. On count 1, rebound in air while raising right leg sideward right; at same time, raise left arm sideward left. On count 2, return to starting position.

Figure 6.6

Freddie
While hopping on right foot, bring left foot forward, touching heel to floor. Hop again on right foot, and bring left foot back to original position.

Repeat action with right foot while hopping on left; opposite arm swings forward.

Figure 6.7

Hop kick
Hop on right leg and kick left leg forward. Hop on left leg and kick right leg forward.

Figure 6.8

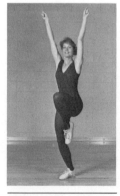

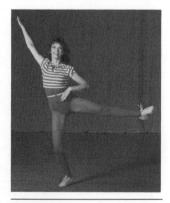

Figure 6.5
Hop with Knee Lift

Figure 6.6
Fly-Away

AEROBIC DANCE

Variations		Safety Precautions
High Level	Low Level	
Swing both arms high overhead then down in front of body on each knee lift. Hop high into air.	Step right and lift knee forward and up.	Land softly on rebound.
Travel sideward on each rebound. Increase height of arm and leg swings.	Step on right foot, raise left leg sideward left. Repeat left.	Land softly after each rebound.
Increase height of arm swings. Kick leg high in front of body.	Step on right foot. Touch left heel to floor in front of body. Swing arms forward. Repeat left.	
Increase height of kick, alternately swinging arms high overhead.	Step on right foot, lift left foot forward. Repeat by stepping on left foot and lifting right foot forward.	Hold to support for balance.

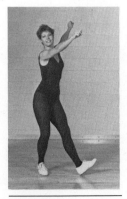

**Figure 6.7
Freddie**

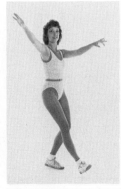

**Figure 6.8
Hop Kick**

Table 6.1   Soft-Rebound Skills Continued

Skills

Jumping jacks
   Count 1: Jump in air and land with feet apart and hands together overhead.

   Count 2: Return to starting position.

Figure 6.9

Rocking horse
   Put weight on left foot, right foot off floor in front of body. In a rocking action forward, transfer weight to right foot. Repeat forward and backward, transferring weight from left to right foot, either 1-count or 2-count rebound with each transfer of weight. To change directions, swing left leg forward and right leg backward.

Figure 6.10

Heel-toe touch
   Count 1: Rebound on left foot and touch right heel to floor.

Figure 6.11a

   Count 2: Rebound on left foot and touch right toe to floor.

Figure 6.11b

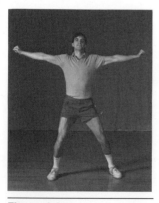

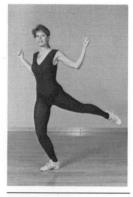

**Figure 6.9
Jumping Jacks**

**Figure 6.10
Rocking Horse**

AEROBIC DANCE

	Variations	
High Level	Low Level	Safety Precautions
	Keeping feet close to floor, alternately lift left leg left and right leg right sideward on each rebound.	*Do not* land with feet farther apart than the width of shoulders. To do so will place strain on knee and ankle joints.
Increase intensity, total body rocking forward and backward with increased height of leg lift.	Step on left foot while lifting right foot forward; step on right foot and lift left foot backward.	
Rebound on left foot, and do a heel-toe touch in succession with right foot. Repeat on right foot with heel-toe touch with left foot. Increase height of rebound and arm swing.	Step with alternate heel touch and toe touch. (Step right heel touch left, step left toe touch right.)	Perform with a soft contact to the floor.

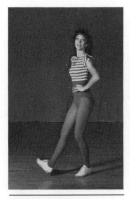

Figure 6.11a
Heel-toe Touch

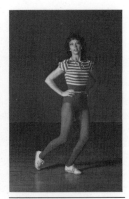

Figure 6.11b
Heel-toe Touch

Soft-Rebound Skills

Table 6.1   Soft-Rebound Skills Continued

Skills

Seat kicker
  Run with opposite heel lifted to buttocks on each step while you perform the arm movements listed in Chapter 4.
Illustration shows back slapper.

Figure 6.12

High knee run
  Run with knees lifted alternately in front of body while you perform each arm movement listed in Chapter 4.
This illustration shows the arm press.

Figure 6.13

Hip swivel
  Count 1: With weight on balls of feet, swivel heels inward.

  Count 2: Swivel heels outward. Make counter rotation with the shoulders.

Figure 6.14

Grasshopper
  On count 1, jump in air then land on left foot; at same time, extend right leg sideward and touch right foot to floor. On count 2, rebound in air, landing with feet together. Arms move out sideward on count 1 and into center of body on count 2.

Figure 6.15

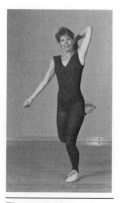 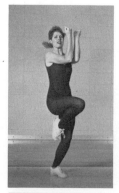

Figure 6.12   **Figure 6.13**
Seat Kicker   **High-Knee Run**

AEROBIC DANCE

| Variations | | |
High Level	Low Level	Safety Precautions
Run with high intensity and vigorous arm movements.	Walking in place, lift opposite foot back and up toward seat.	
Use higher knee lift with "macho" arm movements.	Run, trying to lift knee up. Practice arm actions; 8 reps. each.	Land softly on floor. *Do not* lift feet any higher than allows you to make contact with the floor softly.
Repeat counts 1 and 2, increasing emphasis on twist at waist. Add a high kick on counts 3 and 4.	As you swivel to right with hips, rotate upper body to right also.	Avoid twisting vigorously until completely warmed up.
Move with high intensity. Land with feet crossed at ankles on count 2.	Step on right foot and touch heel of left. Move arms out and in on each step. Repeat left.	

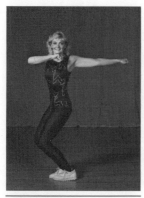

**Figure 6.14
Hip Swivel**

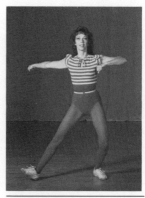

**Figure 6.15
Grasshopper**

Table 6.1   Soft-Rebound Skills Continued

Skills

Whistle-stop jump
  Progress sideward right with series of jumps (legs together, knees bent),
  right arm in air executing a pulling action on each jump, left arm on left hip.

Figure 6.16

Grapevine
  Progress sideward right: (1) step sideward with right foot, (2) step behind
  with left foot, (3) step sideward right, (4) kick left leg forward. Repeat left action progressing sideward left.

Figure 6.17

Scissor run
  Run in place; on count 1, extend nonsupport right leg behind and swing
  right arm upward in front of right shoulder. On count 2, extend left leg behind and swing left arm upward in front of shoulder.

Figure 6.18

Flea hop
  The flea hop is a continuous skipping action. On count 1, hop with right foot,
  moving toward the left; on count 2, hop with left foot, moving to right.

Figure 6.19

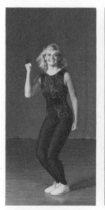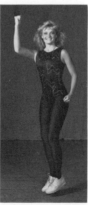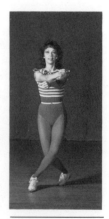

Figure 6.16
Whistle-Stop Jump

Figure 6.17
Grapevine

AEROBIC DANCE

| | Variations | |
High Level	Low Level	Safety Precautions
Increase intensity and vigor of each movement.	Step-together-step sideward right, making pulling action with arms. Repeat sideward. Figure 6.16b	Land lightly on resilient surface.
Select a more vigorous skill, e.g., chorus line kick.	Perform as described without cross step.	
Increase intensity with height of rebound and vigorous arm movement.	Move arms alternately up and down in front of body while lifting alternate leg back and upward.	
Increase height of each skip. Perform 4 hops in sequence in each direction.	Perform sunshine skips.	

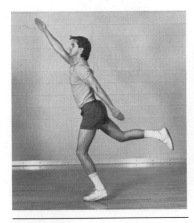

**Figure 6.18
Scissor Run**

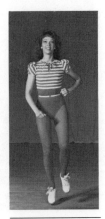

**Figure 6.19
Flea Hop**

Soft-Rebound Skills

Table 6.1   Soft-Rebound Skills Continued

Skills

Chorus line kick

On count 1 (1) hop on right foot while bringing left knee high into center of body.

Figure 6.20a

On count 2 (2) hop on right leg while kicking left leg high in center of body. Hold arms sideward shoulder height. Repeat same action with right leg while hopping on left foot.

Figure 6.20b

Sunshine skip

As you skip on left leg, bring right leg forward and opposite arm forward.

Figure 6.21

Chug

With feet together and knees bent, make successive jumps forward and back in any direction. Bend arms at elbows and swing forward and backward.

Figure 6.22

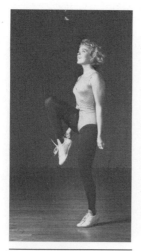

Figure 6.20a
Chorus Line Kick

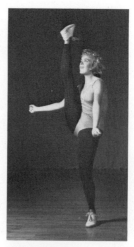

Figure 6.20b
Chorus Line Kick

AEROBIC DANCE

Variations		
High Level	Low Level	Safety Precautions
Increase height of leg kick and knee lift. Increase the number performed in succession.	Lift leg only as high as you can maintain balance.	Warm up the muscles with sustained stretching of hamstrings, quadriceps, heel cord, and ankles.
Increase intensity by higher skip, higher leg lift, and arm swing.	Keep skipping action close to floor and arm swings waist high.	Maintain a fluid motion with a soft rebound.
Alternate with jumping jacks or pendulum steps.	Move body in forward-and-back action by bending and straightening knees.	Practice soft landing on each contact with floor.

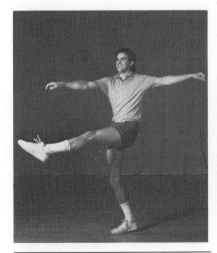

Figure 6.21
Sunshine Skip

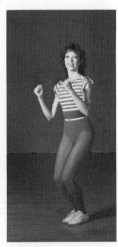

Figure 6.22
Chug

Soft-Rebound Skills

Table 6.1   Soft-Rebound Skills Continued

Skills

Pony

Do a step-ball change-step pattern with the feet. (Raise knees high in air on each change of weight.) Alternately raise one arm high overhead and down to side.

Figure 6.23

Guitar

With strumming guitar action, hop 4 counts right. Repeat hopping to left.

Figure 6.24

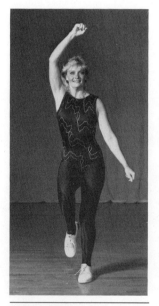 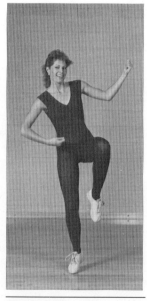

Figure 6.23
Pony

Figure 6.24
Guitar

AEROBIC DANCE

Variations		Safety Precautions
High Level	**Low Level**	
Increase height of knee lift and vigor of arm swing.	Perform a step-to-gether-step-foot pattern alternately raising one arm high, the other arm low.	
Increase intensity with more vigorous movement.	Mimic guitar playing action while doing a step-together-step sideward.	

Table 6.2 Advanced Soft-Rebound Skills and Additional Aerobic Routines

---

Skills

Toe touch

Rebound from left foot to right, and at same time touch left toes to floor. Repeat with rebound to left foot and touch right toes to floor.

Figure 6.25

Boxer shuffle

Make short, quick movements with feet. Shadow box with hands.

Figure 6.26

Rock step

Elbows bent and held close to sides, move body diagonally forward right with rocking motion; feet move forward: step right, close left, step right, hop; on hop, turn diagonally forward left and repeat.

Figure 6.27

Monkey

In gorilla position, slide 2 ×, right hop on count 3, lifting knee high and wide. Arms move up and down alternately in front of body.

Figure 6.28

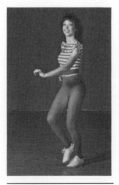 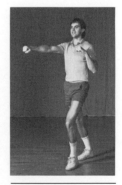

Figure 6.25
Toe Touch

Figure 6.26
Boxer Shuffle

Variations		
High Level	Low Level	Safety Precautions
Increase height of rebound and add high arm swings.	Step on left foot and touch toes of right foot to floor. Repeat by stepping on right foot and touching toes of left foot to floor.	Touch toes lightly to floor. Hold to support, if necessary, for balance.
Increase height of rebound and involve total body in dodging and punching forcefully with hands.	Step on left foot. At same time punch right hand forward. Repeat on right foot while punching forward with left hand.	Perform while seated on straight-back chair.
Clap hands high overhead. Increase height of hop; move body vigorously and with intensity.		
Increase intensity with more vigorous movement.	Mimic arm action while moving sideward with a step-together-step foot pattern.	

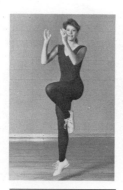

**Figure 6.27
Rock Step**

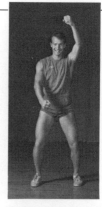

**Figure 6.28
Monkey**

*Table 6.2   Advanced Soft-Rebound Skills and
            Additional Aerobic Routines*

Skills

Ski jumps
  Legs close together, knees bent in downhill ski position, jump from side to side. Raise alternate arm shoulder high.

Figure 6.29

Hopscotch
  On count 1, rebound in air, landing on both feet in stride position. On count 2, rebound in air landing on right foot. Swing left foot behind; touch left foot with right hand. Repeat sequence for count 1; on count 2, rebound in air, landing on left foot while swinging right foot behind.

Figure 6.30

Jester run
  Run in place, lifting free foot to knee of weight-bearing leg, right knee angled sideward right. Touch right foot with left hand.

Figure 6.31

Scissor jump
  Count 1: Rebound in air and land with right leg forward and left leg back.

  Count 2: Rebound in air and land with left leg forward and right leg back. Arms swing opposite to feet.

Figure 6.32

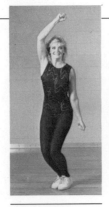

**Figure 6.29
Ski Jumps**

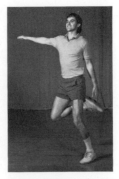

**Figure 6.30
Hopscotch**

AEROBIC DANCE

Variations		Safety Precautions
High Level	**Low Level**	
Jump higher in air on each rebound. Tuck knees to chest on each rebound. Increase counter twist of hips and shoulders.	Select alternate skills such as hip swivel, chug.	Perform only on resilient surface.
Increase intensity of movements.	Step left, swing right leg behind, and touch foot with left hand; repeat by stepping right and swinging left leg behind and touching foot with right hand.	
Run, bringing knee high on each count and touching alternate foot with hand.	Perform a step-hop, lifting alternate foot forward.	Practice soft landing on each contact with floor.
Increase rebound and arm swing.	Move arms alternately up and down in front of body; slide feet alternately forward and back with a slight rebound from floor.	Land with a soft contact to the floor. Keep knees bent throughout.

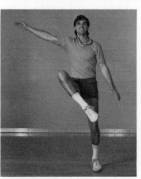

Figure 6.31
Jester Run

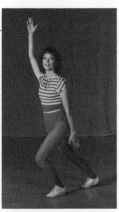

Figure 6.32
Scissor Jump

Soft-Rebound Skills

*Table 6.2   Advanced Soft-Rebound Skills and
            Additional Aerobic Routines*

Skills

High kick

Hop on right foot while kicking left leg waist high; hop on left foot while kicking right leg waist high.

Figure 6.33

Coordination kick

On count 1, rebound in air and land with feet apart; clap hands overhead.

Figure 6.34a

On count 2, rebound in air and land with feet together; hands slap sides of thighs. On count 3, kick right leg high and clap hands underneath.

Figure 6.34b

On count 4, rebound in air and land with feet together; slap hands to sides of thighs. Repeat above, but on count 3, kick left leg high and clap hands underneath.

Hand shadow coordination

While hopping 4 × on right foot, touch left foot in front, side left, front, and back to closed position to change weight. Hands follow same pattern as left foot: front, side, front, down to slap front of thighs. Repeat same action with right foot while hopping on left foot 4 times.

Figure 6.35

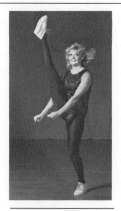

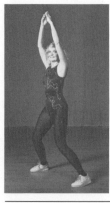

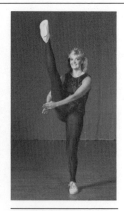

**Figure 6.33
High Kick**

**Figure 6.34a
Coordination Kick**

**Figure 6.34b
Coordination Kick**

AEROBIC DANCE

| Variations | | |
High Level	Low Level	Safety Precautions
Hop on right foot while kicking left leg as high as possible. Clap hands together under the kicking leg.	Perform a step kick forward. Clap hands together in front.	Warm up thoroughly with sustained stretching of hips, legs, feet, and ankles.
Increase intensity and vigor of each movement.	Select alternate skills, such as step kick or step hop.	Do not land with feet farther apart than shoulder width. To do so places stress on ankle and knee joints.
Increase height of the hop. Swing arms overhead as you continue the described leg patterns.	Move arms and left leg in front-side-front-down pattern while standing on right foot. Repeat pattern while standing on left foot.	Warm up hips, legs, and feet with sustained stretching prior to performing this skill.

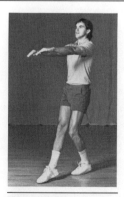

**Figure 6.35
Hand Shadow
Coordination**

Table 6.2   Advanced Soft-Rebound Skills and
Additional Aerobic Routines

Skills

Step-ball-change
  Step on right foot, momentarily shift weight to ball of left foot, and back to
  right foot. Repeat action by starting on left foot.
  Var: Cross right foot in back of left, and momentarily shift weight to ball of
  left foot and back to right.

Figure 6.36

Jump kick
  On count 1, rebound in air, land on both feet. On count 2, rebound in air and
  at same time kick right leg forward. Repeat this sequence, landing on right
  foot on count 2 while kicking left leg forward.

Figure 6.37

Hitch step
  Bend forward at hips; with weight on right foot, take a backward sliding
  hop; repeat with weight on left foot. (Body moves in place. Alternate arm
  swing.)

Figure 6.38

Ski hops
  Assume one-leg tuck position. Hop alternately on right and left foot while
  lifting opposite knee to tuck position.

Figure 6.39

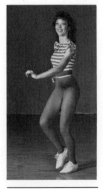 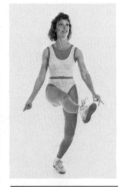

Figure 6.36   Figure 6.37
Step-Ball Change Jump Kick

AEROBIC DANCE

| Variations | | Safety Precautions |
High Level	Low Level	
Do high knee lift and arm swings.	Mimic arm action while moving sideward with step-to-gether-step foot pattern.	
Increase intensity with higher rebound, higher leg swing, and arm swings.	Choose an alternate skill, such as step kick.	Thoroughly warm up feet, ankles, legs, and hips.
Increase intensity with vigorous arm movements and high hop backward.	Step on right foot, lift left knee up. Swing arms alternately. Repeat left.	Contract muscles of abdomen on backward sliding action.
Increase vigor of each action.	Select alternate skill, such as step hop with knee lift.	Perform on resilient surface. Warm up with sustained stretching prior to performance.

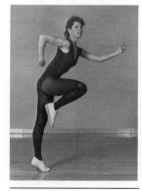

**Figure 6.38
Hitch Step**

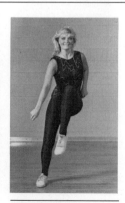

**Figure 6.39
Ski Hops**

Soft-Rebound Skills

Table 6.2   *Advanced Soft-Rebound Skills and*
            Additional Aerobic Routines

Skills

Heel clicks
  Raise right leg sideward right, rebound from left foot, and click heels together side right. Repeat to left side.

Figure 6.40

Sunburst
  Jump in air, spreading legs wide, arms in **V** position overhead.

Figure 6.41

Tuck jump
  Jump in air, bringing knees in tuck position in front of body.

Figure 6.42

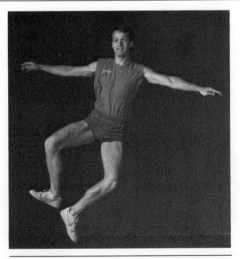

Figure 6.40
Heel Clicks

	Variations		
	High Level	Low Level	Safety Precautions
	Increase height of rebound.	Choose an alternate skill, such as step with a kick forward or heel touch to side.	Perform only on resilient surface. Do not rebound any higher than allows you to land lightly on floor. Thoroughly warm up feet and ankles before performance.
	Increase height of rebound. Also increase number of rebounds in succession.	Choose an alternate skill.	Perform only on resilient surface; wear appropriate soled shoes. Do not rebound any higher than allows you to land lightly.
	Increase height of rebound, height of tuck, and number performed in succession.	Choose an alternate skill, such as step or hop with knee lift.	Perform only on resilient surface. Do not rebound higher than allows you to land lightly.

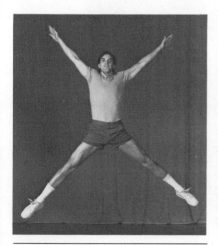

Figure 6.41
Sunburst

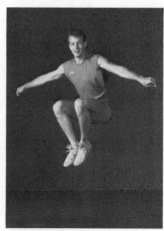

Figure 6.42
Tuck Jump

Soft-Rebound Skills

*Table 6.2   Advanced Soft-Rebound Skills and
             Additional Aerobic Routines*

Skills

Pike jump
  Jump in air, bringing both feet forward from hips and both arms forward.

Figure 6.43

Airborne stride jump
  Jump in air, bringing legs to wide-stride position. Reach hands to feet.

Figure 6.44

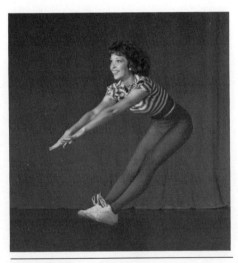

**Figure 6.43
Pike Jump**

AEROBIC DANCE

| Variations | | Safety Precautions |
High Level	Low Level	
Increase height of rebound and extent of pike.	Select alternate skill.	Perform only on resilient surface. Wear appropriate cushion soled shoes.
Increase intensity and height of rebound. Increase number performed in succession.	Select alternate skill, such as jester run.	Perform only on resilient surface and with appropriate shoes. Thoroughly warm up with sustained stretching prior to performance.

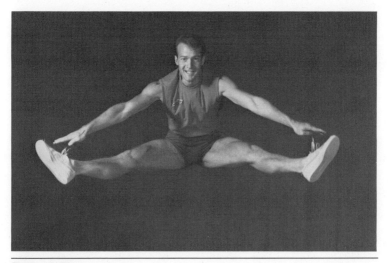

**Figure 6.44
Airborne Stride Jump**

The routines described in this chapter are available on cassette with music and verbal instruction. They are also available on video. See Appendix C.

Routine 6.1

Suggested Music: "Rock-a-Billy"
Style: Soft Rebound
Choreographer: Bard Hill

Seq	Reps	Skills Medium Level	Music Count	Variations High Level	Variations Low Level
Intro	24	Run in place	24	High knees	Foot tread
I	3	3 step hops to right corner with sunshine arms	6	High kick	Step kick Moving forward and backward
	3	3 step hops diagonally back	6		
	6	Repeat 1 × to left corner	12		
II	12	Cowboy kick	24	High side kick	Step, touch heel diagonally forward
I and II		Repeat	48		
Interlude	12	Knee lifts	24	Extend arms overhead and hop high	Step with knee lift.
	2	Flyaway 3 rt 3 left	32		
Interlude		Repeat	24		
I and II		Repeat seq I and II	48		
III	12	Freddie	24	Extend heel off floor	Heel touch on floor
II and III		Repeat seq II and III	48		
I and II		Repeat seq I and II to end of music	84		

Routine 6.2

Suggested Music: "Phunky A"
Style: Soft Rebound
Choreographer: Courtney Ekins

Seq	Reps	Skills — Medium Level	Music Count	Variations — High Level	Variations — Low Level
I	1	Step kick, step kick, jumping jack, push back	8	Use vigorous swings and high kicks	Step touch
		Repeat 5 ×	40		
II	1	Rocking horse: double, double, single, single, single	8		
		Repeat	8		
III	1	Slide right 3 ×, knee lift on count 4.	4	Rebound high in air on the slides.	Walk forward 3 steps, lift left knee. Repeat
		Slide left 3 ×, knee lift on count 4.	4		
II	3	Rocking horse; double, double, single, single, single, single	24		
III	1	Slide right 3 ×, knee lift on count 4. Slide left 3 ×, knee lift on count 4.	8		
II	1	Rocking horse: double, double, single, single, single, single	8		
IV	8	Jumping jack, heel touch, knee lift, high kick	64		
I	8	Repeat I	64		
III	4	Repeat III	32		
V	8	Run forward	8		
	8	Ski jump back	8		
		Repeat routine from beginning or begin Routine Phunky B.			

Routine 6.3

Suggested Music: "People"
Style: Soft Rebound
Choreographer: Courtney Ekins

Seq	Reps	Skills Medium Level	Music Count	Variations High Level	Low Level
I	4	Cowboy kicks	8	Use vigorous arm movements and lift legs high	Step touch
	8	Pendulum swings	8	Use vigorous arm movements and lift legs high	Step touch
		Repeat 3 ×	64		
II	4	Run right 4 counts, jumping jack 2 × while making turn right. Repeat 4 ×, forming a square pattern.	32	Lift knees high	Walk
			32	Lift knees high	Walk
	4	Repeat turning left.			
III	1	Knee lifts 4 right, 4 left	16		
	2	Knee lifts 2 right, 2 left	16		
	4	Knee lifts 1 right, 1 left	16		
IV	8	Jumping jacks	16	Move with high intensity	Step touch
	8	Seat kicker run/circle arms forward	16		
	8	Knee lift run/circle arms backward	16		
	8	Hips swivel/rainbow arms	16		
V	8	Grasshopper	16		
	8	Step kick	16		
	8	Flyaway			
	2	4 right, 4 left	32		
	2	2 right, 2 left	16		
	4	1 right, 1 left	16		
		Repeat II	64		
		Repeat I	16		

Routine 6.4

Suggested Music: "Up-N-At-Em"
Style: Soft Rebound
Choreographer: Claudia Hill

Seq	Reps	Skills Medium Level	Music Count	Variations High Level	Low Level
Intro	1	Whistle-stop jump, 4 right, 4 left	8	Travel to left and right	Step touch sideward
Interlude	4	Step kick	8		right, 8 ×.
Intro	1	Whistle-stop jump, 4 right, 4 left	8		Repeat 1, 8 ×, repeat
I	2	2 knee lifts left leg, 2 right	4	High knee lift	Step lift without hop
	1	Grapevine left	4	High kick on beat 4	Touch on beat 4
	3	Repeat right–left–right	24		
II	2	2 twosies, starting left leg	4	High kick to side	Keep one foot on floor while raising other sideward. Repeat on alternate side.
	4	4 pendulum swings	4		
		Repeat 3 ×	24		
I	2	2 knee lifts right	4	High knee lift	Step lift without hop
	1	Grapevine	4	High kick on beat 4	Touch on beat 4
	3	Repeat right–left–right	24		
III	4	Freddie	8	Extend heel off floor vigorous arms	Step and touch front
	4	Scissor Run	8	Extend legs back and high	Step and touch back
	2	Repeat 2 ×	16		

Soft-Rebound Skills

Routine 6.4 (Continued)

Seq	Reps	Skills Medium Level	Music Count	Variations High Level	Variations Low Level
Intro	2	Whistle-stop jump, 4 right, 4 left	8		
	2	Repeat	8		
I	4	Knee lift and grape-vine seq	32		
II	4	Twosie and pendu-lum seq	32		
III	8	Repeat 2 ×	64		
Interlude	2	Chorus kick	8	High kick	Step kick
	8	Flea hop	8	High knees	Eliminate hop
	3	Repeat 3 ×	48		
Intro	2	Whistle-stop jump, 4 right, 4 left	8		
	2	Repeat	8		
I		Repeat	64		
II		Repeat 2 ×	64		

Routine 6.5

Suggested Music: "Hooked on the 50's"
Style: Soft Rebound
Choreographer: Claudia Hill

Seq	Reps	Skills — Medium Level	Music Count	Variations — High Level	Variations — Low Level
Intro	32	Swivel hips	32	Place arms above head	
I	4	Sunshine skip: forward diagonally	8	Use high kick	Heel touch
	4	right, backward to original position.	8		
	4	Forward diagonally	8		
	4	left, backward to original position.	8		
II	4	Hop kick right (guitar step)	8	Travel farther with a high hop and kick	Shuffle sideward instead of hop
	4	Hop kick left (guitar step)	8		
	4	Hop kick right (guitar step)	8		
	4	Hop kick left (guitar step)	8		
III	2	Chug right and left	4	Apply high energy	Omit turn
	4	Swivel hips, turning ¼ to right	4		
		Repeat 3 × to make a square	24		
IV	16	Pony	32	Lift knees high	Triple step
		Repeat I, II, III, IV	128		
		Repeat I, II, III, IV	128		
		Repeat I, II	64		

Routine 6.6

Suggested Music: "Hooked on Aerobics"
Style: Soft Rebound
Choreographer: Kent Streuling

Seq	Reps	Skills Medium Level	Music Count	Variations High Level	Variations Low Level
Intro		Running in place	16	Lift knees high	Heel touches
I		Jumping jack, knee lift right	4	Extend arms up in air	Heel touch instead of knee lifts
		Jumping jack, knee lift left	4		
		Alternate knee lift 4 ×; right, left	8		
		Repeat	16		
II	1	Jumping jack, knee lift right	8	Perform jumping jack in air	Smooth impact, no bouncing
		Jumping jack, knee lift left			
III	8	Step kick forward	16	Kick leg up high	Low impact, no bouncing
I	2	Repeat	32		
II		Repeat	8		
III		Repeat	16		
IV	3	4 runs, 2 jumping jacks (moving right)	48	Perform with high knees and jumping jack in air	Stay in place, low impact
		Repeat (moving left)			
I	2	Repeat	32		
II		Repeat	8		
III		Repeat	16		
IV		Repeat	48		
V	2	Knee lifts in 4s (4 on right, 4 on left)	32	Move across floor	No bouncing, low knee lifts
	16	Step kick forward	32	High kicks	No bouncing, low kicks
IV	4	Repeat	64		
I	4	Repeat	64		
III	To end	Repeat			

AEROBIC DANCE

Routine 6.7

Suggested Music: "Phunky B"
Style: Soft Rebound
Choreographer: Colleen Anderson

Seq	Reps	Skills Medium Level	Music Count	Variations High Level	Low Level
I	32	Twist in place; swing arms at various levels	32	Swing arms high overhead	Keep arms low, easy twist
II	2	Travel right and left with twist; clap on count 8 each time	32	Travel as far as possible on twist	Stay in place on twist
III	4	2 kicks, forward right; repeat left 4 twists in place Freddie right and left Repeat	64	Do high kicks, exaggerated movement on twists and Freddies	Use low kicks, easy twist, easy Freddies
IV	4	4 run to side right, 1 jumping jack, 1 knee lift right Repeat opposite direction	64	Travel on runs, high knee lift	Use easy runs, low knee lift
V	1	Knee lift right, Freddie left, 4 × Knee lift left, Freddie right, 4 ×	16 16	Lift knees high, exaggerate movement on Freddies	Use low knee lift, easy movement on Freddie
I		Repeat	32		
II		Repeat	32		
III		Repeat	64		
IV		Repeat	64		

Routine 6.8

Suggested Music: "High Energy"
Style: Soft Rebound
Choreographer: Kent Strueling

Seq	Reps	Skills Medium Level	Music Count	Variations High Level	Low Level
Intro	6	Run in place 4 counts	52	High knees	Heel touches
I	2	Run, run, step, hop right Run, run, step, hop left (clap on hops)	16	High hops, high knees	Step in place Step with alternate knee lift
	8	Cowboy kicks	16	High kicks	Heel touches
		Repeat	32		
II	2	Knee lifts (4 right, 4 left)	16	High kicks	Step with alternate knee lift
	8	Freddies	16	High kicks	Step kick
	10	Knee lifts	20	High kicks	Heel touches
I	2	Repeat	32		
II	8	Knee lifts	16		
	8	Freddies	16		
	8	Knee lifts	16		
III	8	Jumping jack, chug	32	Extend high and rebound high	Low level jumping jack
	16	Step kick front	32	High kicks	Heel touches
I		Repeat 2 ×	32		
II	8	Knee lifts	16		
	8	Freddies	16		
	8	Knee lifts	16		

Injury, Stress, and Pain: Prevention and Cure

A common misconception held by poorly qualified instructors and participants in physical fitness programs is that "If it isn't hurting, it isn't working." Pain is the body's only way of warning a participant that the activity must be modified or physical damage will result. Often the enthusiasm and encouragement of the instructor, the enjoyment of performing aerobic routines to up-beat music, and the competitive spirit of "keeping up" with the group sets an atmosphere conducive to ignoring stress, strain, and pain until a disabling injury results.

Because of the ballistic nature of many aerobic dance programs and the number of times the feet make contact with the floor, there is a great deal of stress and trauma to the feet, the lower extremities, and often the back. This stress and trauma can be minimized by following these basic rules:

1. Wear shoes that provides a good arch support, a firm heel support, and support for lateral movement and that have a smooth, cushioned sole.
2. Perform on resilient surfaces. Tile, cement, or any other nonresilient surface does not provide a good performance facility. The best surface is wood on a raised spring frame.

Most Frequent Aerobic Dance Injuries

More than 90 percent of the injuries resulting from aerobic dance occur below the knees. The most common injury is shin splints, followed by knotted muscles in the calf. A high percentage of aerobic instructors suffer from overexercised muscles and joint trauma. The recommended time limit for aerobic dance workout is thirty minutes. It is also recommended that you not participate in high-intensity, impact-style aerobics on consecutive days.

Exercises to Avoid

This section describes commonly performed exercises that bring stress and trauma to the joints of the body. The photographs depict improper performance. The pain marks (″″) on the photographs indicate the area of stress and trauma. The dotted lines and arrows indicate necessary corrections. The *Do Not* is a recommendation that these exercises be eliminated from your workout.

1. Avoid movements that result in pressure at an angle to the weight bearing surface. For example, when performing jumping jacks, if you land with your feet farther apart than shoulder width, you place undue stress at the ankle and knee joints. See Figure 7.1.
2. The knee joint is a hinge joint; any twist, turn, or lateral pressure can result in injury to the connective tissue (ligaments, tendons, and cartilage). See Figures 7.2–7.4.
3. Avoid exercise that places undue tension on the discs between the vertebrae of the spinal column. See Figures 7.5–7.7.

Even in the most carefully designed and conducted aerobic fitness programs, participants may experience pain, strain, or other abnormal stress. Study Table 7.1 to learn how to prevent exercise-related injury, recognize symptoms, and respond with proper treatment.

Column one in Table 7.1 describes common symptoms, and column two identifies possible causes. Column three gives procedures you should take to prevent the injury. The fourth column recommends treatment procedures to follow.

CPR (cardiopulmonary resuscitation) training is available in most communities in the United States. Take advantage of this training and become qualified to act prudently in case of accident or injury.

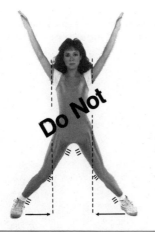

Figure 7.1 Avoid exercise that places pressure at an angle to the weight-bearing surface

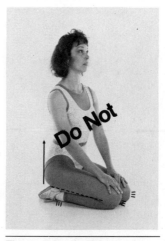

Figure 7.2 Avoid exercise that brings the calf and the back of the thigh together.

Figure 7.3 Avoid exercise that places lateral pressure on the knee.

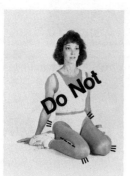

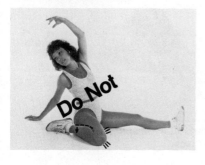

Figure 7.4 Perform with center of knee joint in line with ankle bone and center of hip to avoid hyperextension of knee joint.

Injury, Stress, and Pain

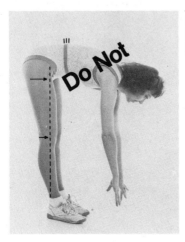

Figure 7.5 When bending forward, keep knees bent to avoid stress on posterior longitudinal ligament.

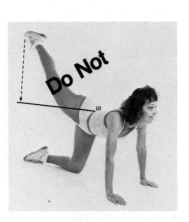

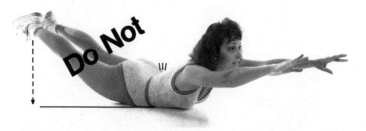

Figure 7.6 Avoid twisting in the forward bent position.

Figure 7.7 Avoid movements that force the spinal column out of alignment, placing stress on the discs.

AEROBIC DANCE

Table 7.1   Prevention and Treatment of Exercise-Related Injury and Stress

Symptoms	Causes	Prevention	Treatment
Abnormal heart action: Irregular pulse, palpitation of chest and throat, sudden burst of rapid heartbeat, sudden very slow pulse following rapid pulse	Overstress (may or may not be dangerous)	Consult physician and follow prescribed program.	**Stop activity.** Immediately consult physician and follow prescribed program.
Pain or pressure in center of chest, arm, or throat precipitated by or following exercise	Possible heart pain due to stress	Consult physician and follow prescribed program.	**Stop activity.** Consult physician and follow prescribed program.
Dizziness, light-headedness, cold sweat, glassy stare, pallor, fainting, blueness	Insufficient blood to the brain	Consult physician and follow prescribed program.	**Stop activity.** Consult physician and follow prescribed program.
Flare-up of arthritic condition or gout	Trauma to joints, usually hips, knees, ankles	1. Follow lower level of conditioning. 2. Wear cushion-soled shoes. 3. Exercise on resilient surface. 4. Follow proper warm-up.	1. Rest. Do not resume exercise until condition subsides, then resume at lower level. 2. Follow procedures recommended by physician. 3. Prescribe conditioning exercise that puts less strain on specified joints.

Table 7.1   Prevention and Treatment of Exercise-Related Injury and Stress

Symptoms	Causes	Prevention	Treatment
Nausea or vomiting after exercise	Not enough oxygen to the intestines. Exercising too intense or cool-down too quick.	Exercise at lower level of your PTZ or below.	Exercise less vigorously; keep moving at a slower pace after exercise until heart rate is near normal.
Side ache (stitch in the side); sticking feeling under the ribs while exercising.	Spasm of the diaphragm (large muscle separating chest from abdomen) or lack of oxygen or buildup of carbon dioxide (trapped gas)	Use a proper warm-up, not progressing too fast. Slow down, breathe properly.	Slow down. Forcefully exhale on each breath. While sitting, lean forward, attempting to push the abdominal organ up against the diaphragm.
Blisters	Separation of layers of skin caused by rubbing against nonyielding surfaces. Buildup of fluid.	Wear properly fitted shoes. Wear two pairs of socks. Cover area with Vaseline. Use talcum powder.	Ice hot spots when they first appear. Apply ice 10 min., 20 min. maximum. Drain fluid. Cover with medicated ointment. Use doughnut-shaped pad made from moleskin and foam.
Muscle soreness and stiffness	Lack of strength in given muscle. Lack of proper stretching and warm-up. Progression level and intensity too high. Start exercise program slowly and progress gradually.	Follow progressive resistance exercises for strength; do at lower level. Follow progressive resistance exercises for flexibility; do at a lower level. Perform stretching with a sustained, continuous movement.	May require complete rest or change to a lower level of activity. Apply ice packs (10–20 min.), then stretch. Do slow, gradual stretching of muscles (avoid overstretching). *(Continued on p. 99.)*

Table 7.1   Prevention and Treatment of Exercise-Related
            Injury and Stress

Symptoms	Causes	Prevention	Treatment
Muscle soreness and stiffness *(continued)*	Jerking, bobbing, or bouncing on stretched muscle. Exercising on hard surfaces.	Wear thick-soled shoes with arch support. Perform on soft surface, such as grass, wood, carpet, mat.	If muscle soreness persists, use ice packs for 3 days. Then use moist heat (packs, whirlpool) to warm-up with stretch. Ice after activity with stretch.
Painful arch	Usually caused by wearing improperly fitting shoes, being overweight, or performing on hard surfaces.	Properly fitted shoes with cushioned soles. Go on weight-reduction program with proper level of activity, i.e., walking program prior to dancing, jogging, running, etc.	Proper shoes, resilient surfaces. Hydrotherapy (warm foot bath, whirlpool). Proper conditioning program for foot.
Muscle fatigue	Muscles have not been properly conditioned before vigorous activity.	Proper conditioning. Less strenuous activity.	Stretch with slow, sustained action. Ice packs and stretch. Follow progressive resistance program within PTZ.
Shinsplints (pain along anterior portion of lower leg)	Inflammation of connective tissue between bones in lower leg or muscle. Activity too vigorous; improper conditioning. Improperly fitting shoes; overweight.	Wear shoes with thicker soles; proper arch support. Work out on resilient surface. Follow proper conditioning program.	Properly fitted shoes with arch supports, possibly with raised heel. Proper conditioning, including stretching the muscle. Workouts must be on resilient surface.

Table 7.1   *Prevention and Treatment of Exercise-Related Injury and Stress*

Symptoms	Causes	Prevention	Treatment
Tendonitis	Overstretching of Achilles tendon resulting in inflammation.	Proper heel-cord stretch prior to workout, followed by ice, massage. Pushing heel to floor on each landing from a jump or hop.	Use moist heat before workout. Perform sustained stretch. Apply ice after activity, repeat sustained cord stretch.
Sprain	Injury to ligament caused by abnormal range of movement in joint. Ligament may be stretched, partially torn or completely torn. Abnormal range of movement can be caused by landing wrong on floor, twisting, or being hit.	Follow progressive resistance program. Strengthen each muscle group.	Ice, compression, elevation, medical attention.
Stress fracture—pinpoint pain during activity and sometimes when at rest. Swelling may be present.	Jarring and jolting during activity.	Proper shoes. Proper conditioning. Perform activity on soft surface.	Reduce or eliminate activity. Seek medical attention. When in doubt (1) RICE (Rest and apply ice packs) and (2) seek medical attention.

Appendix A
Physical Fitness Assessments

Appendix A will help you determine your present fitness level and show you how you rank against predetermined norms. It will also help you establish goals that are realistic for you to achieve and provide charts for you to monitor your progress.

You can find out how fit you are by taking the tests for muscular strength and endurance, tests for flexibility, cardiovascular tests, and body composition assessment described in this appendix.

Preparation

1. You will need this equipment:
    Clock or stopwatch with a second hand.
    Ruler, yardstick, or measuring tape.
    Bench 15 inches high for men, 13 inches high for women.
2. Have a partner work with you to complete each test as described. Record the results on the Personal Assessment Chart (PAC) (Figure A.1)
3. Write your name and age on the Personal Assessment Chart.
4. After performing each of the tests, record the date and your score in column I. **Note:** In approximately six weeks, take the same tests again, recording the date and the scores in column II. You should follow the same procedures every six weeks so that you can see your progress as you move to a higher level of fitness.

Determining General Characteristics

Height. Remove your shoes. Measure your height while standing against a wall. Record it in feet and inches.

Body Frame. To approximate the size of your body frame, measure the width of your elbow (Figure A.2). If you have a caliper, use it to measure the space between the two prominent bones on either side of your elbow. You can also measure the distance between the two bones with a ruler. Compare this measurement with measurements for medium-framed men and women (Table A.1). Measurements less than

Physical Fitness Assessments   101

Figure A.1   Personal Assessment Chart (PAC)

Name _____

ID No. _____

Age _____   Sex M F   Height _____   Body Frame _____

	I	II	III	IV
Date	_____	_____	_____	_____
RHR	_____	_____	_____	_____
Cardiovascular fitness				
5-min. step test	_____	_____	_____	_____
1.5 mile run	_____	_____	_____	_____
Flexibility				
Shoulders	L __ R __	L __ R __	L __ R __	L __ R __
Hamstring	_____	_____	_____	_____
Lateral stretch (side bend)	L __ R __	L __ R __	L __ R __	L __ R __
Strength				
Push-ups (circle level 1, 2, or 3)	1 2 3	1 2 3	1 2 3	1 2 3
Abdominal curls (circle level 1, 2, or 3)	1 2 3	1 2 3	1 2 3	1 2 3
Body fat Caliper test (skinfold measure)	_____	_____	_____	_____

Address: _____

_____

Phone: _____

those listed indicates that you have a small frame. Higher measurements indicate a large frame.

Weight. Remove your shoes and outer clothing. Weigh yourself on standardized scales that will be available each time you record your weight. Record your weight on the PAC chart, Figure A.1. Compare your weight with information listed in Table A.2.

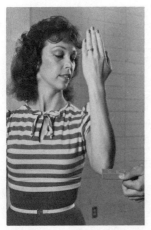

**Figure A.2
Measuring the Body Frame**

Table A.1   Measurements for Medium-Frame Men and Women

Height in 1" heels Men	Elbow Breadth	Height in 1" heels Women	Elbow Breadth
5'2"–5'3"	2½"–2⅞"	4'10"–4'11"	2¼"–2½"
5'4"–5'7"	2⅝"–2⅞"	5'0"–5'3"	2¼"–2½"
5'8"–5'11"	2¾"–3"	5'4"–5'7"	2⅜"–2⅝"
6'0"–6'3"	2¾"–3⅛"	5'8"–5'11"	2⅜"–2⅝"
6'4"	2⅞"–3¼"	5'0"	2½"–2¾"

Resting Heart Rate. The resting heart rate (RHR) measures how hard your heart works (beats per minutes) to sustain the body systems while you are at complete rest. To monitor your RHR, count your heartbeats for *one minute* while *lying down* after at least a two-hour rest or sleep. A convenient time for taking your RHR is just before getting out of bed after a night of sleep. You need a watch or clock clearly visible from your bed to eliminate movement before monitoring your heart rate.

You can best find your pulse on your wrist approximately one and one-half inches above the thumb joint. You can also find your pulse on your neck along the side of your voice box, one-half inch below the jaw

Table A.2 1983 Metropolitan Height and Weight Tables

MEN

Height Feet	Inches	Small Frame	Medium Frame	Large Frame
5	2	128–134	131–141	138–150
5	3	130–136	133–143	140–153
5	4	132–138	135–145	142–156
5	5	134–140	137–148	144–160
5	6	136–142	139–151	146–164
5	7	138–145	142–154	149–168
5	8	140–148	145–157	152–172
5	9	142–151	148–160	155–176
5	10	144–154	151–163	158–180
5	11	146–157	154–166	161–184
6	0	149–160	157–170	164–188
6	1	152–164	160–174	168–192
6	2	155–168	164–178	172–197
6	3	158–172	167–182	176–202
6	4	162–176	171–187	181–207

WOMEN

Height Feet	Inches	Small Frame	Medium Frame	Large Frame
4	10	102–111	109–121	118–131
4	11	103–113	111–123	120–134
5	0	104–115	113–126	122–137
5	1	106–118	115–129	125–140
5	2	108–121	118–132	128–143
5	3	111–124	121–135	131–147
5	4	114–127	124–138	134–151
5	5	117–130	127–141	137–155
5	6	120–133	130–144	140–159
5	7	123–136	133–147	143–163
5	8	126–139	136–150	146–167
5	9	129–142	139–153	149–170
5	10	132–145	142–156	152–173
5	11	135–148	145–159	155–176
6	0	138–151	148–162	158–179

Courtesy of Metropolitan Life Insurance Company. Copyright 1983.

Source of basic data 1979 Build Study Society of Actuaries and Association of Life Insurance Medical Directors of America 1980.

bone or over the temple in front of your ear. Monitor your heartbeat by lightly placing two or three fingers along the artery on your wrist, your temple, or your throat and counting the beats for one minute. Do not use your thumb to monitor your pulse. (The thumb has its own pulse.)

Follow this procedure on three different days to verify the results. Average the scores (add the three scores and divide by three).

Example: day 1 _____ , day 2 _____ , day 3 _____
Total of day 1, 2 and 3 = _____ divided by 3 = RHR score _____ .
Record this number on your PAC.

Muscular Strength and Endurance Assessment

Muscular strength and endurance are vital to an aerobic conditioning program. Often you are unable to achieve an aerobic training effect simply because your muscles become fatigued before the intensity and duration criteria are met.

Strength is defined as the capacity of a muscle to exert maximal force against a resistance. *Muscle endurance* is defined as the capacity to exert force repeatedly over a period of time. Strength and endurance are interrelated and are prerequisite to all facets of movement, health, and well-being. Correct body alignment, efficiency and grace in movement, and success in performing recreational and life-enrichment skills depend on muscular strength and endurance.

Also, the higher your ratio of lean body mass (muscle tissue) to fat body mass, the higher your metabolic rate. With a strength and endurance training program, resulting in increased lean body mass, and thus an increase in metabolic rate, the end result is a more efficient use of caloric energy. This phenomenon allows the person with a greater percent lean body mass to consume more calories each day while maintaining a healthy percent body fat. We have already learned that muscles atrophy if not used, resulting in less lean body mass, and, consequently, a decrease in metabolic rate.

Muscle strength and endurance should be assessed before you engage in a physical conditioning program so that proper training can be prescribed and monitored. The following tests are recommended to assess strength of the arms (pushups) and the abdominal muscles (curl-ups). Three levels of each test provide a base from which almost any participant can perform at least one repetition. The tests follow the principals on which conditioning is based; thus, you are able to repeat the test in your daily fitness program.

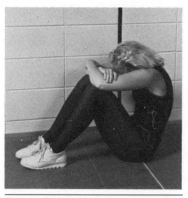

Figure A.3
Abdominal Curls, Level 1

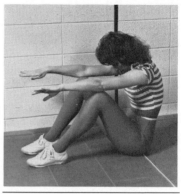

Figure A.4
Abdominal Curls, Level 2

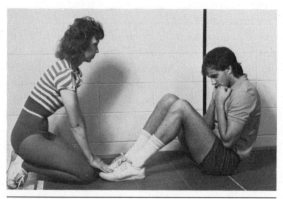

Figure A.5
Abdominal Curls, Level 3

TEST 1 FOR MUSCULAR STRENGTH AND ENDURANCE:
ABDOMINAL CURLS

Directions: Assume one of the positions illustrated in Figures A.3–A.5, knees bent, feet flat on the floor 12 to 18 inches from buttocks, with a partner giving light support to hold feet in contact with the floor.

Record the number of times you are able to perform a sit-up done by curling the upper torso and bringing the shoulders to a 90° angle with the hip joint. In level 3, your arms must be held tightly to your body. Return to starting position, upper back touching floor between each count. Select one of the three levels; perform at the highest level you can with a slow, controlled, continuous action. Your score is the number of curls you can do without stopping. Record your score in the appropriate space provided on your PAC and circle the level at which you performed.

TEST 2 FOR MUSCULAR STRENGTH AND ENDURANCE: PUSHUPS

Assume one of the positions shown in Figures A.6–A.8. Perform at the highest level possible for you. Record the number of times you are able to touch your chin to the floor and return to starting position. Record the number in the space provided on your PAC, and circle the level at which you performed.

Flexibility Assessment

Flexibility is defined as the range of motion at each joint of the body. Range of motion is determined by the elasticity of surrounding muscles.

PRETEST WARMUP

You are able to score higher on flexibility assessments after an aerobics workout. According to research conducted at Brigham Young University in the aerobic dance program, participants scored higher on the flexibility tests and did not suffer posttest strain or stiff muscles when following a prescribed program of (1) a preliminary warm-up, (2) a 10- to 15-minute aerobics workout within their personal training zone, and (3) a posttest cool down. (See warm-up and cool-down exercises in Chapter 3.)

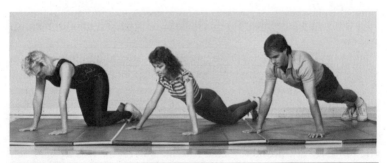

| **Figure A.6** | **Figure A.7** | **Figure A.8** |
| **Pushups, Level 1** | **Pushups, Level 2** | **Pushups, Level 3** |

Physical Fitness Assessments

TEST 1 FOR FLEXIBILITY: SHOULDER GIRDLE

Directions: While in a standing position, reach your right arm back over your right shoulder and the left arm under the left shoulder (Figure A.9). Try to touch your fingertips together. If you are unable to touch your fingertips, have your partner measure the distance between the third finger of your hands; record that distance with a minus sign (−) on your PAC. If you are able to overlap your fingers, measure the distance of your overlap and place a plus sign (+) by that number. Record the results in the space by "R" on the PAC. Repeat the same test with the left arm reaching over the left shoulder and the right arm reaching under the right shoulder. Record this score in the space by "L" on the PAC. Record the best score of three attempts each for right (R) and left (L).

TEST 2 FOR FLEXIBILITY: HAMSTRING AND LOWER BACK MUSCLES

Necessary equipment: A surface six inches off the floor with a measuring scale clearly marked at one-half inch increments from a restraining board.

Directions: For the sit-and-reach test (Figure A.10), remove shoes and sit with both feet flat against the restraining board approximately shoulder width apart. With a slow sustained movement, reach directly forward with hands on top of one another, palms down. You can have three tries reaching along the measuring scale; hold the position of maximum reach for one second. Both hands must be at the same distance for the test to be valid.

TEST 3 FOR FLEXIBILITY: LATERAL STRETCH (SIDE BEND)

Necessary equipment: Smooth-surfaced wall and ruler or measuring tape.

Directions: Stand with your shoulders, back, and hips against the wall and your feet approximately twelve inches apart (Figure A.11). Bend sideways at the waist and reach your hand down the side of your leg. Be sure to keep your shoulders, back, and hips against the wall and both feet flat on the floor. Your knees must remain straight. Have a partner measure the distance from your fingers to the floor. When all the above criteria are met, record this distance on the PAC as you reach to the left side to measure right side flexibility and again as you reach to the right side to measure left side flexibility.

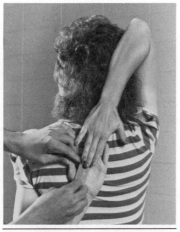

Figure A.9
Shoulder Girdle Flexibility Test

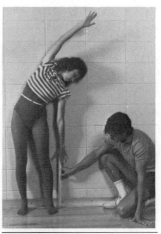

Figure A.11
Lateral Stretch

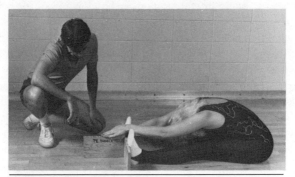

Figure A.10
Hamstring and Lower Back Flexibility Test

Cardiovascular Fitness Assessments

Cardiovascular fitness is the ability of the heart and lungs to supply needed blood and oxygen to the muscles while they perform work during an extended period of time.

You can score higher on cardiovascular fitness tests and not suffer posttest ill effects if you (1) do not engage in any vigorous aerobic activity before the tests and (2) prepare your body for the assessment by a pretest warm-up.

SUGGESTED PRETEST WARM-UP

1. Light exercises of walking and treading feet while swinging arms to increase circulation to all muscles.
2. Sustained stretching of major muscle groups: shoulders, torso, lower back, hamstring, front of thigh, tibialis anterior and posterior, calf, and heel cord. (See directions in Chapter 3.)

STEP TEST
(SUBMAXIMAL TEST TO PREDICT CARDIOVASCULAR FITNESS)

Necessary equipment: Bench or stool (15 inches for men, 13 inches for women); stopwatch with second hand; metronome or musical recording of 90 beats per minute.

Preparation: You and your partner should practice taking your pulse to ensure accuracy. One of you should monitor your pulse on the wrist and the other along the voice box or temple.

For a warm-up, see the suggested warm-up for "Cardiovascular Fitness Assessment.")

Directions: Begin by stepping up on and down from the bench or chair (see Figure A.12). On beat one, step up on one leg; on beat two, step up with the other leg; on beat three, step down with one leg; on beat four, step down with the other leg. Continue this procedure for five minutes. At the end of five minutes, sit down for fifteen seconds.

During this 15-second rest, you and your partner should each find your pulse, one at the throat, the other on the wrist (Figure A.13). At the end of this 15-second rest, both you and your partner count the pulse for 15 seconds on the signal from the timer. Compare the heart rates to validate the score. If you have a discrepancy of more than four beats, retake the test on a subsequent day. This is your post-pulse score.

Refer to Tables A.3 and A.4, and find your post-exercise pulse count in the left column. Follow across the table until you are in line with your nearest body weight, as indicated in pounds across the top of the table. This figure is your weight-adjusted fitness level. Find your age-adjusted fitness score in Table A.5 by following across the table till you are in line with your nearest age. Record this score on your PAC.

Use tables A.6 and A.7 to find your present cardiovascular fitness level.

Note: You are disqualified if you are unable to step 90 times a minute for the full five minutes. But do not give up if you are unable to complete the test this time. Start a walking program, or begin your aerobic dance program at level one and then test yourself in three or four weeks

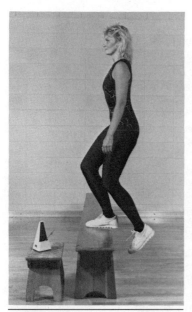

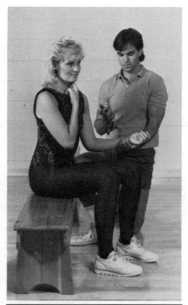

Figure A.12
Step Test

Figure A.13
Measuring Pulse After Step Test

or as soon as you are able to complete the test according to the specifications.

After completing the assessment, do not sit or lie down until you have had a proper cool-down.

Suggested Cool-Down: Jog or walk slowly until your heart rate slows down to near normal. Or repeat the sustained stretching warm-up exercises illustrated in Chapter 3.

ONE AND ONE-HALF MILE RUN

The one and one-half mile run is a maximal test to predict cardiovascular condition. But it is recommended only for persons who have been preconditioned by following an aerobic program and have attained the "good" level as assessed by a submaximal test such as the step test or walk/run test.

Necessary equipment and facility: Stop watch and a measured 1.5 mile distance on appropriate surface.

Directions: The timer will start the watch as you take off from the designated starting line. Run or walk, trying to cover the distance in

Table A.3 Fitness Score for Men

BODY WEIGHT

	120	130	140	150	160	170	180	190	200	210	220	230	240	
45	33	33	33	33	33	32	32	32	32	32	32	32	32	45
44	34	34	34	34	33	33	33	33	33	33	33	33	33	44
43	35	35	35	34	34	34	34	34	34	34	34	34	34	43
42	36	35	35	35	35	35	35	35	35	35	35	34	34	42
41	36	36	36	36	36	36	36	36	36	36	36	35	35	41
40	37	37	37	37	37	37	37	37	36	36	36	36	36	40
39	38	38	38	38	38	38	38	38	38	38	38	37	37	39
38	39	39	39	39	39	39	39	39	39	39	39	38	38	38
37	41	40	40	40	40	40	40	40	40	40	40	39	39	37
36	42	42	41	41	41	41	41	41	41	41	41	40	40	36
35	43	43	42	42	42	42	42	42	42	42	42	42	41	35
34	44	44	43	43	43	43	43	43	43	43	43	43	43	34
33	46	45	45	45	45	45	44	44	44	44	44	44	44	33
32	47	47	46	46	46	46	46	46	46	46	46	46	46	32
31	48	48	48	47	47	47	47	47	47	47	47	47	47	31
30	50	49	49	49	48	48	48	48	48	48	48	48	48	30
29	52	51	51	51	50	50	50	50	50	50	50	50	50	29
28	53	53	53	53	52	52	52	52	52	52	51	51	51	28
27	55	55	55	54	54	54	54	54	54	53	53	53	52	27
26	57	57	56	56	56	56	56	56	56	55	55	54	54	28
25	59	59	58	58	58	58	58	58	58	56	56	55	55	25
24	60	60	60	60	60	60	60	59	59	58	58	57		24
23	62	62	61	61	61	61	61	60	60	60	59			23
22	64	64	63	63	63	63	62	62	61	61				22
21	66	66	65	65	65	64	64	64	62					21
20	68	68	67	67	67	66	66	65						20
	120	130	140	150	160	170	180	190	200	210	220	230	240	

POST-EXERCISE PULSE COUNT

as short a time as possible. The timer will stop the watch as you cross the finish line. Record the time on your PAC. Refer to Tables A.8 and A.9 to find your age-adjusted fitness rating.

Body Composition Assessment

The body is made up of lean body tissue and fat tissue. Bones, muscles, and internal organs make up what is referred to as lean body mass. Fat tissue is commonly referred to as fat mass or percent body fat.

Table A.4   Fitness Score for Women

BODY WEIGHT

POST-EXERCISE PULSE COUNT	80	90	100	110	120	130	140	150	160	170	180	190	
45										29	29	29	45
44								30	30	30	30	30	44
43							31	31	31	31	31	31	43
42			32	32	32	32	32	32	32	32	32	32	42
41			33	33	33	33	33	33	33	33	33	33	41
40			34	34	34	34	34	34	34	34	34	34	40
39			35	35	35	35	35	35	35	35	35	35	39
38			36	36	36	36	36	36	36	36	36	36	38
37			37	37	37	37	37	37	37	37	37	37	37
36		37	38	38	38	38	38	38	38	38	38	38	36
35	38	38	39	39	39	39	39	39	39	39	39	39	35
34	39	39	40	40	40	40	40	40	40	40	40	40	34
33	40	40	41	41	41	41	41	41	41	41	41	41	33
32	41	41	42	42	42	42	42	42	42	42	42	42	32
31	42	42	43	43	43	43	43	43	43	43	43	43	31
30	43	43	44	44	44	44	44	44	44	44	44	44	30
29	44	44	45	45	45	45	45	45	45	45	45	45	29
28	45	45	46	46	46	47	47	47	47	47	47		28
27	46	46	47	48	48	49	49	49	49	49			27
26	47	48	49	50	50	51	51	51	51				26
25	49	50	51	52	52	53	53						25
24	51	52	53	54	54	55							24
23	53	54	54	56	56	57							23
	80	90	100	110	120	130	140	150	160	170	180	190	

According to a study by the National Institutes of Health (NIH) of the U.S. Public Health Service, obesity is a killing disease that should receive the same medical attention as high blood pressure, smoking, and other physical disorders that cause serious illness and premature death. The study noted that any level of obesity increases health risks, but the level of 20 percent or more above "desirable" body weight was the point at which doctors should treat an otherwise healthy adult. Health problems that the NIH attributed directly to obesity were high blood pressure, high blood cholesterol, adult-onset diabetes, several types of cancer, heart disease, gall bladder disease, menstrual abnormalities, respiratory problems, and arthritis. It was also noted that "the enormous psychological burden may be the greatest adverse effect of obesity."

Table A.5 Age-Adjusted Scores

	NEAREST AGE											
	15	20	25	30	35	40	45	50	55	60	65	
30	32	31	30	29	27	26	25	24	23	22	21	30
31	33	32	31	30	28	27	26	25	24	23	22	31
32	34	33	32	31	29	28	27	26	25	24	23	32
33	35	34	33	32	31	30	29	28	27	25	24	33
34	36	35	34	33	32	31	30	29	28	26	25	34
35	37	36	35	34	33	32	31	30	29	27	26	35
36	38	37	36	35	34	33	32	31	30	28	27	36
37	39	38	37	36	35	34	33	32	31	30	28	37
38	40	39	38	37	36	35	34	33	32	31	29	38
39	41	40	39	38	37	36	35	34	33	32	30	39
40	42	41	40	39	38	37	36	35	34	33	31	40
41	43	42	41	40	39	38	37	36	35	34	32	41
42	44	43	42	41	40	39	38	37	36	35	33	42
43	45	44	43	42	41	40	39	38	37	36	34	43
44	46	45	44	43	42	41	40	39	38	37	35	44
45	47	46	45	44	43	42	41	40	39	37	36	45
46	48	47	46	45	44	43	42	41	40	38	37	46
47	49	48	47	46	45	44	43	42	40	39	38	47
48	50	49	48	47	46	45	44	43	41	40	38	48
49	51	50	49	48	47	46	45	44	42	41	39	49
50	53	51	50	49	48	47	46	45	43	42	40	50
51	54	52	51	50	49	48	47	45	44	42	41	51
52	55	53	52	51	50	49	48	46	45	43	42	52
53	56	54	53	52	51	50	49	47	46	44	42	53
54	57	55	54	53	52	51	50	48	46	45	43	54
55	58	56	55	54	53	52	51	49	47	46	44	55
56	59	57	56	55	54	53	52	50	48	46	45	56
57	60	58	57	56	55	54	52	51	49	47	46	57
58	61	59	58	57	56	55	53	52	50	48	46	58
59	62	60	59	58	57	55	54	53	51	49	47	59
60	63	61	60	59	58	56	55	53	52	50	48	60
61	64	62	61	60	59	57	56	54	53	51	49	61
62	65	63	62	61	60	58	57	55	53	51	50	62
63	66	64	63	62	60	59	58	56	54	52	50	63
64	67	65	64	63	61	60	59	57	55	53	51	64
65	68	66	65	64	62	61	60	58	56	54	52	65
66	69	67	66	65	63	62	61	58	57	55	53	66
67	70	68	67	66	64	63	62	59	58	56	54	67
68	71	69	68	67	65	64	63	61	59	57	54	68
69	72	70	69	68	66	65	64	61	59	57	55	69
70	74	71	70	69	67	66	65	62	60	58	56	70
71	75	72	71	70	68	67	65	63	61	59	57	71
72	76	73	72	71	69	68	66	64	62	60	58	72

FITNESS SCORE

The NIH also found that the distribution of fat deposits, as indicated by a high ratio of waist to hip circumference, is associated with a higher risk for illness and decreased life span. It has been estimated that if obesity were eliminated, the average life span could increase by as much as five years. Obesity is also highly correlated with accidental death rate. The increase in mortality with relative weight is more dramatic with a long duration of obesity.

IDEAL FAT BODY MASS

Fat tissue is essential: it insulates the body against the elements, helps protect the internal organs from shocks and blows to the body, and provides the storage for energy needs and fat-soluble vitamins A, D, E, and K. A person needs only enough fat tissue to meet these essentials.

Reliable research indicates that women should carry approximately 17 to 20 percent body fat, and men should carry approximately 12 to 15 percent. People who eat to provide the needed daily nutrients and work or exercise at extremely high energy levels can maintain excellent health with a lower percentage of body fat.

Research indicates that people who are underweight fall into categories of poor health and well-being relative to the degree of malnourishment and percent essential fat. The lower limits of essential fat

Table A.6 Physical Fitness Rating for Men

(*Use age-adjusted score*)

Nearest Age	Superior	Excellent	Very Good	Good	Fair	Poor	Very Poor
15	57+	56–52	51–47	46–42	41–37	36–32	31–
20	56+	55–51	50–46	45–41	40–36	35–31	30–
25	55+	54–50	49–45	44–40	39–35	34–30	29–
30	54+	53–49	48–44	43–39	38–34	33–29	28–
35	53+	52–48	47–43	42–38	37–33	32–28	27–
40	52+	51–47	46–42	41–37	36–32	31–27	26–
45	51+	50–46	45–41	40–36	35–31	30–26	25–
50	50+	49–45	44–40	39–35	34–30	29–25	24–
55	49+	48–44	43–39	38–34	33–29	28–24	23–
60	48+	47–43	42–38	37–33	32–28	27–23	22–
65	47+	48–42	41–37	36–32	31–27	26–22	21–

Table A.7   Physical Fitness Rating for Women

(*Use age-adjusted score*)

Nearest Age	Superior	Excellent	Very Good	Good	Fair	Poor	Very Poor
15	54+	53–49	48–44	43–39	38–34	33–29	28–
20	53+	52–48	47–43	42–38	37–33	32–28	27–
25	52+	51–47	46–42	41–37	36–32	31–27	26–
30	51+	50–46	45–41	40–36	35–31	30–26	25–
35	50+	49–45	44–40	39–35	34–30	29–25	24–
40	49+	48–44	43–39	38–34	33–29	28–24	23–
45	48+	47–43	42–38	37–33	32–28	27–23	22–
50	47+	46–42	41–37	36–32	31–27	26–22	21–
55	46+	45–41	40–36	35–31	30–26	25–21	20–
60	45+	44–40	39–35	34–30	29–25	24–20	19–
65	44+	44–39	38–34	33–29	28–24	23–20	19–

Tables A.3 through A.7 reprinted from Sharkey, Brian J., *Physiology of Fitness,* by permission of publishers, Human Kinetics, 1979, Champaign, IL.

needed to maintain good health are 5 percent for men and 10 percent for women. Lower percentages place the individual in a high-risk category for illness and decreased life span.

ASSESSMENT TECHNIQUES

A great deal of research has been conducted to try to determine the most accurate procedures for assessing the percent of fat body mass and lean body mass of an individual. There is no simple, objective, and truly accurate method of measurement for a living person. However, several methods can be used to estimate fat and lean body mass. Select one of the following methods.

Skinfold thickness method. In the skinfold method, the skin and the fatty tissue between the skin and muscle are pinched and measured. Based on the estimation that 50 percent of the fatty tissue in the body is deposited directly under the skin, a fairly accurate measurement can be made.

Skinfold calipers. Calipers are made by many companies and range in styles from hand-controlled, pressure-operated tools to computer-programmed scientific instruments. The prices vary according to the sophistication of the instrument. But the validity and reliability of the measurement depends on the technician. Most colleges and fitness

Table A.8   1.5 Mile Test

	Ratings for Men			
Fitness Category	Under 30	30–39	40–49	50 +
I. Very Poor	16:30 +	17:30 +	18:30 +	19:00 +
II. Poor	16:30–14:31	17:30–15:31	18:30–16:31	19:00–17:01
III. Fair	14:30–12:01	15:30–13:01	16:30–14:01	17:00–14:31
IV. Good	12:00–10:16	13:00–11:01	14:00–11:31	14:30–12:01
V. Excellent	<10:16	<11:01	<11:31	<12:01

Table A.9   1.5 Mile Test

	Ratings for Women			
Fitness Category	Under 30	30–39	40–49	50 +
I. Very Poor	17:30 +	18:30 +	19:30 +	20:30 +
II. Poor	17:30–15:31	18:30–16:31	19:30–17:31	20:30–18:31
III. Fair	15:30–13:01	16:30–14:01	17:30–15:01	18:30–16:31
IV. Good	13:00–11:16	14:00–12:01	15:00–12:31	16:30–13:31
V. Excellent	<11:16	<12:01	<12:31	<13:31

centers have instruments and trained technicians. Manufacturing companies provide specific instructions for use as well as predetermined equation charts. The calipers provide a scientific approach to the pinch-an-inch method and has become the most popular technique used for assessing body composition. To ensure reliable measurements, pretests and posttests should be administered by a reliable, trained technician, and the test should be administered in the morning before vigorous exercise.

Suggested Readings

Books

Arnheim, Daniel D. *Dance Injuries: Their Prevention and Care.* St. Louis: C. V. Mosby Company, 1980.

Arnheim, Daniel D. *Modern Principles of Athletic Training.* St. Louis: Times Mirror/Mosby College Publishing, 1985.

Herrscher, Michelle Welch. *Forever Fit.* Salt Lake City: Deseret Book Company, 1985.

Hoeger, Werner W. K. *Lifetime Physical Fitness and Wellness.* Englewood, Colorado: Morton Publishing Company, 1986.

Jacobson, Phyllis C., and Ann Valentine. *Fundamental Skills in Physical Education.* Provo: Brigham Young University Press, 1977.

Jacobson, Phyllis C., and Barbara Vance. *Move It! Proven Exercises for Family Health and Fitness.* Salt Lake City: Bookcraft, Inc., 1978.

Jensen, Clayne R., and A. Garth Fisher. *Scientific Basis of Athletic Conditioning.* Philadelphia: Lea & Febiger, 1972.

Katch, Frank I., and William D. McArdle. *Nutrition, Weight Control, and Exercise.* Philadelphia: Lea & Febiger, 1983.

Miller, David K., and T. Carl Allen. *Fitness: A Lifetime Commitment.* Minneapolis: Burgess Publishing Company, 1979.

Thomas, Tom R., and Carole J. Zebas. *Scientific Exercise Training.* Dubuque: Kendall/Hunt Publishing Company, 1984.

U.S. Department of Health and Human Services. *The Health Consequences of Smoking—Cancer and Chronic Lung Disease in the Workplace.* A Report of the Surgeon General, 1985.

Periodicals

Bale, P., E. Colley, and J. L. Mayhew. "Relationships Among Physique, Strength, and Performance in Women Students." *Journal of Sports Medicine,* 25 (1985): 98–103.

Blyth, Michelle, and Brian R. Goslin. "Cardiorespiratory Responses to 'Aerobic Dance.'" Studies and Researches. *Journal of Sports Medicine,* 25 (1985): 57–64.

Burton, Benjamin T., and Willis R. Foster. "Health Implications of Obesity: An NIH Consensus Development Conference." *Perspectives in Practice,* 85 (September 1985): 1117–1121.

Claremont, Alan D., Sandra A. Simonwitz, Marie A. Boarman, Ann O. Asbell, and Steven J. Auferoth. "The Ability of Instructors to Organize Aerobic Dance Exercise into Effective Cardiovascular Training." *The Physician and Sportsmedicine,* 14, No. 10 (October 1986): 89–100.

Cullumbine, H. "Relationship Between Body Build and Capacity for Exercise." *Journal of Applied Physiology* Vol. 2 (September 1949): 155–168.

Davis, Paul O., Charles O. Dotson, and Arthur V. Curtis. "A Simplified Technique for the Determination of Per Cent Body Fat in Adult Males." *Journal of Sports Medicine,* 25 (1985): 255–261.

Gossard, Denis, William L. Haskell, C. Barr Taylor, J. Kurt Mueller, Flay Rogers, Margaret Chandler, David Ahn, Nancy H. Miller, and Robert DeBusk. "Effects of Low- and High-Intensity Home-Based Exercise Training on Functional Capacity in Healthy Middle-Aged Men." *The American Journal of Cardiology,* 57 (February 15, 1986): 446–449.

Marwick, Charles. "Campaign Seeks to Increase US 'Cholesterol Consciousness.'" *Medical News,* 255, No. 9 (March 7, 1986): 1097–1102.

Parachini, Allan. "New Aerobics Guidelines Announced by Women's Health Care Specialists." *Los Angeles Times,* 6 May, 1986: Part V, pp. 1, 4, 5.

Schlife, John E. "Fitness Testing in Family Practice." *The Physician and Sportsmedicine*, 10, No. 10 (October 1982): 142–154.

Solomon, Ruth L., and Lyle J. Micheli. "Technique as a Consideration in Modern Dance Injuries." *The Physician and Sportsmedicine*, 14, No. 8 (August 1986): 83–89.

Stamford, Bryant. "Testing Your Aerobic Fitness." *The Physician and Sportsmedicine*, 13, No. 2 (February 1985): 194.

The Stanford University Heart Disease Prevention Program Magazine. (February 1986): 34–64. Rodale Press, Inc.

Watterson, Valerie V. "The Effects of Aerobic Dance on Cardiovascular Fitness." *The Physician and Sportsmedicine*, 12, No. 10 (October 1984): 138–145.

Appendix C
Audio and Video Instructional Materials

Audiocassette

The suggested upbeat music and routines are available on audiocassettes.

"HOOKED ON AEROBICS 90-Minute Cassette"—ALL ORIGINAL MUSIC ($12.95)

Side A. 45 Minutes of Vocal Instruction

Side B. 45 Minutes of Music

Home Video Tapes

"HOOKED ON AEROBICS HOME VIDEO" (Available in VHS or BETA FORMAT)

Vol. I *FITNESS IS FOR EVERY BODY* ($29.95 + $1.50 mailing)
Two aerobic exercise programs (one 40-minute and one 50-minute workout) on a 90-minute tape. Choose your effort level from three levels—low, medium, or high—and then follow the vibrant instructors at your level in your own home.

Vol. II *FITNESS FOR SPECIAL POPULATIONS* ($29.95 + $1.50 mailing)
This 90-minute video presents four separate physical fitness programs. You can follow grandparents, parents, young adults, children, and nonambulatory young men and women on three effort levels of aerobic dance, ball handling, and rope jumping as well as warm-up and cool-down exercises in each program. These programs are designed for physical fitness and skill development in the home, in the school, in the community, and in rehabilitation units and hospitals. Instruction guidelines for parents, teachers, and unit leaders accompany each video.

For ordering materials and for further information regarding workshops and certification clinics write to:

Thompson Productions, 1060 E. 800 S. Orem, UT 84058

Index

(Those entries marked with an asterisk (*) include a photograph of an aerobic dance skill.)

8 4 1 8